Dancing with MySelf

Sensuous Exercises for Body, Mind and Spirit

Katia de Peyer

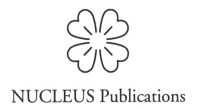

NUCLEUS Publications

Dancing with MySelf
Sensuous Exercises for Body, Mind and Spirit
by Katia de Peyer
Illustrated by Michael B. McClure

Published by NUCLEUS Publications, Rt. 2 Box 49, Willow Springs, MO 65793. Send for free catalog.

Library of Congress cataloging in Publication Data.
Peyer, Katia de. 1933—
    Dancing with MySelf: Sensuous Exercises for Body, Mind and
Spirit / by Katia de Peyer.
        p.   cm.
    Includes index.
    ISBN 0-945934-04-1: $9.95
    1. Exercise. 2. Dancing. 3. Mind and body. 4. Spiritual
formation. I. Title.
GV505.P445   1991
613.7'1--dc20   90-27891
                                                      CIP

Printed in the United States of America

Dauringter Myself

To my daughter

95

$10

K. de Peyer

ACKNOWLEDGMENTS

A very special thanks to Janet Hubbard-Brown for her insightful developmental editing and the enthusiasm with which she came to my help. Her intuitive understanding of the material and her resourcefulness contributed greatly to its clarity.

Many thanks also to all the people who have been part of the process: to Jane Dowd for her great help with the organization of the first three chapters; to Vimala McClure for her encouragement, her patience and for making the book happen; Michael McClure for enlivening the book with his art, to Diane Von Furstenberg for her affectionate encouragement and to Valerie Aubry whose wise guidance during all these years of gestation has provided me with a Northern Star.

TABLE OF CONTENTS

INTRODUCTION

Dancing With MySelf is an intuitive approach to physical fitness which embraces the mind and spirit. Your goal is not only to maintain shape and youthful looks, but to go inward as well, deep inside, to the source of your own renewal. Before change is possible, you must accept yourself as you are.

Your road to self-transformation goes through nine sensuous steps. I have found each one of these steps of great value in maintaining my own vitality and beauty. You will discover that beauty cultivated within reflects without. Each one of these sensuous steps will reveal to you a new way to celebrate life.

Over three centuries ago, the poet John Milton searched for a word that would embody all the senses. It did not exist, so he created the word *sensuous*. Sensuous is often confused with the word *sensual* because both words share the same root, "sense." Although the dividing line between the two seems tenuous, the difference in meaning is significant. Sensuous connotes a state of delight in the sensations of touch, taste, shape, sight, smell and sound. It is the delight of furthering our appreciation of life, of letting our horizons widen as our senses become the missing link between our minds and our soaring spirits! On the other hand, the word "sensual" implies gratification of the sexual impulse. Sensuous opens a new landscape; sensual reduces the experience to a specific activity.

The first five steps take you on an inner journey where you will discover how to become centered and how to build a positive self-image. You will learn how natural breathing is a source of renewal, how to navigate through your daily activities without being consumed by stress, and the wonders of the Law of Polarity. Taking care of yourself comes naturally when you feel centered, secure, and serene, and when you understand the forces—such as gravity and vital energy—that regulate your life.

Steps Six through Eight guide you in taking care of your joints and muscle tone. I use the term "Practice Lab" rather than exercise, which implies physical activity only. It is assumed by many that exercise should be repetitive and strenuous in order to be effective, and that it is okay for the mind to wander, endlessly distracted by mental tapes. People say, "I hate to exercise." I am not surprised; who likes a mechanical activity devoid of meaning? These Practice Labs lead to a sequence of movements flowing beautifully into a dance form. The final chapter leads you into the meditative realm, where you learn to feel at peace with yourself and eventually in harmony with the rest of the world.

My early training as a dancer inspired in me the need to seek and understand the source of beauty. My role models—the great dancers of my youth—dedicated themselves to the art of Terpsichore, the muse of Dance and Song. Yearning to discover her secrets, I soon became aware that accomplished ballet dancers at all times seek within themselves clarity, simplicity, calmness and concentration. This was the beginning of my journey towards self-discovery and trans-formation. Following this path, I have traveled to many places and opened myself to many experiences.

My journey originated in France where I was born. When I was four, my mother enrolled me in ballet school in Paris, and by age 13 I was training seriously alongside some of the major ballerinas of the day. I went on to work in London with Madame Rambert at the Mercury Theater and to study Flamenco later in Madrid with La Quica. (La Quica taught the famous dancer and choreographer Leonide Massine Spanish steps which Massine used when he created his grand master-piece, "The Three-Cornered Hat," which is still in the repertoire of major ballet companies.)

When my training was complete, I danced professionally and then became a movement therapist. I opened a women's movement class in the early sixties at Carita of Paris, an internationally known house of beauty care. For the past 20 years, I have had a private clientele in New York City where I live part of the year.

My purpose in writing this book is to share with you the insights and experiences that I have gleaned from a lifetime of teaching. I have been on an inner journey of self-development which makes me aware of the healing potential we carry within, if only we could have a peek inside ourselves!

The key to a positive life is to discover the divine spark within, to love ourselves first, without which we cannot love our neighbors. I am not speaking of self-indulgence but of respecting, loving, taking good care of the person you are, because you are a manifestation of God's spirit. Not God as a father figure outside yourself, but the God within. The God in your heart encourages you to be one with the spirit within. It demands that you be centered, so that your three planes of expression—mind, body and spirit—become one. What do I mean by spirit? The divine spark as expressed in your intuition, feelings, thoughts and imagination; that which heightens your consciousness and spurs your creativity.

Steps One to Five: The Inner Journey

The first five steps are related to your inner development and lead to the mastery of self. It is not enough to tighten your thighs or flatten your stomach. Your thoughts need discipline in order to understand the different currents of energy which influence your personality and to find new ways to practice wellness in your life. One such modality is visualization—a mental practice using suggestion or imagery directed to specific points in order to cause a change in consciousness. To best use the visualizations given throughout the book, record them on tape and play them back when you can fully relax and let them work with your imagination. Visualizations to be recorded will appear in italics. Read them slowly, pausing for a few moments where indicated.

The word "beingness" is used to convey your essence—that part of you which never changes. It is your own divine nature as opposed to your personality, which you shape, mold and help create with the many decisions you constantly make. The term "in your mind's eye" relates to your imagination as a guide to your feelings. How long has it been since you took the time to know how you feel about yourself? Give it time. You are rediscovering yourself. The universe is not in a hurry. In the words of the Taoist master Lao Tse, "The journey of a thousand miles begins with a single step."

Directions

I suggest you read Step One through to the end, then go back and do the Practice Labs once every day for a week unless otherwise indicated. Only then go to the next step, through Step Five. Practice Labs offer practical experiments or pose questions relating to the text. Questions are there not so much to be answered as to stimulate your thinking. They act as pointers to tell you, "This is the moment to search and discover more about yourself." Allow each question to sit in your mind, so to speak, to have a vibration of its own. Each question is like a flashlight scanning a dark room in order to find the switch. The whole purpose is to illuminate the entire house!

Journal

As you proceed on your inner journey of self-transformation (first five steps), you will keep a journal. Starting with Step One, keep a notebook next to you as you do your second reading. Enter the date and write down with each headline the main points of each experiment as you have done it. Then briefly assess your experience or answer the questions posed. The purpose of your journal is to help you remember what you've accomplished, to keep a record of each experiment, and evaluate your progress as you go along.

The word *Journal* at the end of a paragraph indicates a pause for writing. At the end of each chapter you will find a quiz for your journal relating to the Labs. This is a checkpoint. After doing the quiz you may wish to go over some of the experiments before you continue.

In each of the first few steps you will find a **Tool**. A Tool is a specific experiment that stands out because it encapsulates the essence of that particular step. When you know the Tool well, practice it any time you need to. Each Tool is ideal for use in moments of stress or confusion as each one embodies in a clear and effective way the principles of each step. Each Tool has been chosen for its effectiveness. It is yours for life and as you climb the steps in this book, you are gathering five Tools which comprise your Sensuous Awakening Kit. Describe each Tool in your journal.

When you reach the end of the steps, you can repeat them again and again. Each time you will discover something new about yourself. Your journal will stand by your side like a friend, ready to give you supportive feedback.

Steps Six to Eight: The Outer Journey

The next three steps guide you to take care of your physical self. You will learn the wisdom of warming up to maintain flexibility. You will find that your spine is your most important structure, since every part of you is either supported by or attached to it. You will discover the importance of your pelvic structure in relation to your back. You will learn that each back stretch and abdominal toner contributes to the health of your back since muscles work in tandem.

Your outer journey will take place over five weeks, after which you will use a simpler format to keep you in shape. The first week (Step Six), you begin your journey with a daily Tune-up Program of thirteen limbering movements to be repeated as shown. The second week (Step Seven) you begin your Workout Program, which consists of three sections. These exercises are done daily over the next three weeks: Section A, in the second week, takes care of your back and abdomen. Section B, in the third week, takes care of your limbs. Section C, in the fourth week, helps you learn centering and balance. Simple and easy to do at first, the exercises help you build your Workout Program like pieces of a puzzle. When you get to the fourth week you will have the complete picture—a program which takes only 20 minutes of your time.

The fifth week (Step Eight) you arrive at your daily maintenance program. This is the goal you have been working toward. It is the icing on the cake; I call it the Dance. The Dance is a sequence designed around 88 movements, most of which you already know from your Workout Program. Each movement follows the previous one at an even pace in a way that the sequence becomes a dance. Once you are familiar with it, it will take only about seven minutes. Of all human activities, dancing expresses best the joy of being alive. All creation moves; only human beings have the privilege to dance in celebration of life.

Why do I call it a Dance? Although you will be familiar with some of the movements, in this sequence you practice the art of moving from one figure to the other in a flowing, attentive way. The dance sequence will guide you to the development of your own style. What is style? It is a combination of your own timing which creates what musicians call *phrasing*—attention to details and an overall sensitivity to the line of movement. The sense of completion will come. You will find out when you arrive at the end of the sequence you are already at the beginning again!

Step Nine: Completion

You are back at the beginning. In Chapter One you have practiced centering. Here, the practice is on a higher level. You will practice clearing your mind and attuning to your Higher Self, which is the Divine Spirit within you. "Clearing the Mind" is a mental practice that helps you release anxiety and confusion. It is a centering, soothing method to clear the way for the voice within—your inner guide. "Attuning to the Higher Self" is a practice which attunes you to the unlimited source of love energy within your heart.

Practice, enjoy and work on it! Plant your garden with new seeds. The crop will be plentiful, believe me!

STEP ONE
Discovering Your Center

Have you ever caught your breath while watching a ballet, transported by the extraordinary beauty and grace of the dancers' movements? Dancers, whose bodies communicate to their audience a tale of human action, emotion or spirit, prepare for a performance—and even daily exercise—by centering themselves. For the ballet dancer, the first movement at the barre is a *plie*, which is bending the knees with heels together and toes turned out. This movement is of utmost importance as it gives the performer a chance to establish her mood by getting in touch with the inner self.

If you look at the face of a professional dancer doing a *plie*, you will be amazed by the degree of pure concentration brought to bear on what seems such a simple task! All this concentration is attuned toward the inner self. The dancer listens to the awakening of every tissue, nerve, muscle fiber and breath in order to feel in command of the whole self— to feel centered.

As a young ballet student, I practiced my *plies* with great seriousness. As I matured, I came to understand how our bodies are living instruments which can be fine-tuned by centering our attention. My purpose in this Step is to share this knowledge with you, so that you too can learn how to be in command of your whole self.

Awareness
In your search for center, you need to be increasingly more aware of yourself in relation to the world in which you live. Let me share with you an experience of mine. Positioning myself at the wooden barre as a young ballet student, I discovered that the mere contact of the wood under my hand could give me energy. I noticed this particularly if I was not holding onto it, but merely feeling its contact. It was as though in my preparation for the correct position, the wood under my hand awakened in me the sensation of the outside world as a warm loving support. I was no longer bound by my own skin. I felt extended out into space— no longer alone, but connected.

Practice Lab: Developing Awareness
Stop yourself during the day and notice what you have in your hands.

See if you are able to hold it with just the right amount of energy so you do not grab or squeeze it. Don't let it go. Feel secure in your ability to offer support. Experience the life energy in the object you hold.

As you give the object the chance to rest in your hand, you are allowing your perception of it to stimulate you. It will have a life of its own. It is as though you awaken its energy. Try this again and again. You will be amazed how your attention span widens and what you will discover in the world around you. Be aware of what you are doing and when you are doing it.

Journal: *Without using visual references, describe an object. Use words which capture its feeling and energy.*

Practice Lab: Centering

The head symbolizes thinking and mental activity. The heart symbolizes feeling and spiritual activity. The abdomen signifies visceral and instinctive activity.

Centering is the ability to bring into focus the sum of one's own physical and mental attention. The act of centering prepares you for action, creating a heightened sense of "livingness" within self.

Focus your attention inside your head and close your eyes. Take a few deep breaths and imagine the breath moving to your head. Stay with the experience for a few minutes until the inside of your head feels very alive. Open your eyes. Does it feel like your head is the center of your being? Focus your attention in your chest where your heart is located and open your upper chest to deep breathing. Close your eyes and stay with the experience the same amount of time as before. Open your eyes. Does it feel like your chest is more alive than your head? Direct your attention to your abdominal area and feel your breath moving accordingly. Close your eyes and sense the feeling of being alive in that area.

Each time you direct your attention within your physical self, you become fully present within the confines of that area; you illuminate that area with the full dimension of your being—mental, emotional and spiritual. You become centered. Could you be centered everywhere? Yes! Your whole being, each one of your millions of cells, could be fully alive. You could be perfectly centered like a highly developed yogi or Zen Buddhist. If you are only alive in your head, you are one temperament, and if you are only alive in your abdomen, you are another type of temperament. The idea is to be alive everywhere!

Close your eyes once more. See whether you can feel alive in your head as well as your chest and your abdomen and after a while choose the place where your natural center feels located. You will find it midway between your chest and your abdomen. Your natural center is the place where your breathing moves freely and your focal point of attention feels equidistant between your ground and the top of your head.

Journal: Write about your center. Where is it? What parts of your body feel alive? What parts have little feeling?

Practice Lab: Centers of Perception

When you direct your attention to a particular area of your body, there is an activation of your brain cells and a change in bodily reactions. Each thought has a biochemical component. Each time you focus on one particular area of your body, you have created a center of perception. It feels alive. You have activated a new pathway of interaction between specific brain cells and the cells of the specific physical area.

Set a timer for five minutes. Close your eyes and direct your thoughts to your right hand for several minutes. After a while, you will notice that your right hand feels warmer. Do the same thing with your left hand.

You have experienced 1) awareness of your physical interaction with objects outside yourself and 2) mental awareness within yourself. Now you are to experience awareness on the spiritual level. Remember that the spiritual pertains to the imagination. It is the intuitive faculty of those of us who remember our divine origin. The artist, the poet, the mystic draw inspiration from that inner source where imagination can lead to ecstasy. With practice, you can too!

Practice Lab: Spiritual Center

Close your eyes and focus your attention on your heart. Hold your attention there for a few minutes. Open yourself to the feeling inside. Can you feel your pulse in your heart? Now imagine your heart slowing down, the pulse becoming very quiet. Feel your breathing quiet down and move to your heart. Imagine a white light like candle-light in the center of your heart. Focus on it for a minute or two. Can you see it?

Open your eyes. Are you more aware of your spiritual space?

Test your degree of self-awareness. Is it the world outside which attracts your attention, or is it the inner world which prevails? Give yourself a few minutes to experience the difference.

Journal: Describe your heart-space. What does it look like? What is its texture? How does it feel?

Practice Lab: Inner Space

Many activities happen simultaneously in your inner space: breathing, blood flow, digestion, nerve impulses and endocrine activities. All of this is happening whether you are active or at rest. Have you ever thought about this? How much of this inner functioning can you feel? How much of it do you think you could feel if you were to give it your utmost attention?

Let's try to discover more about you. Close your eyes after each of the following questions. Experience the answer, then write it in your journal.

1) How tall do you feel you are from the top of your head to your feet?

2) How wide do you feel you are through your shoulders? Through your hips?

3) Do you feel as wide through your shoulders as you feel through your hips?

Journal: Take time to sense how you feel in space. Write about it.

Practice Lab: Spine Center

Your spine is the axis which determines the alignment of your whole structure. With eyes closed, visualize your spine. Can you see with your mind's eye the spot right below the skull where the spine originates? Can you feel it? Your spine stretches from that point, which is the first vertical vertebrae, all the way to the sacrum at the base. Can you see the place where it ends? Can you see it in your mind's eye?

Let your mind go slowly down your spine from top to bottom and slowly up again. Repeat this visualization three times a day until you feel familiar with it. What it feels like is the purpose of the practice, not what you *think* it should feel like. Remember, thinking is connected to the head or mind, and feeling is connected to the heart or spirit.

Journal: Describe your spine as it appears to you in this visualization exercise.

Practice Lab: Outer Space

International law relating to territorial waters states that a country can claim a certain amount of sea space off its shores. Couldn't we claim the same for our bodies? Indeed, the space within the reach of our arms and legs can be considered ours.

Begin to develop a sense of skin perception. It is easiest when at the beach where you can feel the sun and air on your skin. When you walk down the street, notice the air against your skin. When it is windy, don't fear it. Offer your skin to the experience rather than resisting it. Do the same with rain. Work with all elements of the weather. How does your skin feel when it is dry? Wet? Allow yourself to perceive shades of difference in the state of your skin. Observe how your awareness is growing.

Journal: Write about one experience you had this week and how it felt to your skin.

Practice Lab: Pendulum (daily for one week)

I call this experiment the 'pendulum'. You experience your outer living space as you move forward, sideways and backwards while your feet are glued to the ground. Every time you return to the vertical position; you find your center. You experience your command over the forces of balance and gravity as well as your ability to adjust yourself to these forces.

1 Place your feet firmly on the ground.
2 Slowly lean forward as one unit, keeping your feet where they are, as far as you can go without losing your balance.
3 Return to the first position, where you feel perfectly straight again. Think of yourself as a vertical line forming a 90 degree angle with the ground.
4 Slowly lean backward (with no break through the hips) as far as you can go without losing your balance.
5 Return to the first position.

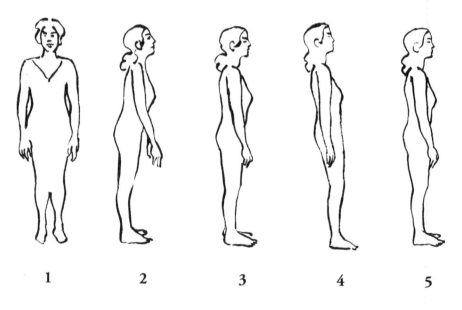

1   2   3   4   5

6 Now the pendulum moves sideways. Shift your weight toward the right as far as you can.

7 Return to the first position.

8 Shift your weight towards the left as far as you can go.

9 Return to where you feel you are no longer fighting gravity.

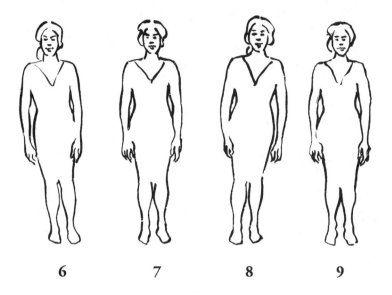

6   7   8   9

The place where you no longer feel the pull of your weight in any direction is the place where your body is in perfect alignment. You feel your spine centered with the ground.

Habits and conditioning pull us outside of ourselves throughout the day. At the office, on the road, watching TV—the world outside demands our attention. How can we respond and yet remain well-balanced and healthy? We have to find our own source of energy. The experience of centering can provide just that.

Practice Lab: Inner and Outer Self (daily for one week)

This experiment brings the imagination into play, as well as increasing awareness. You can find your center as well as align your body with the earth.

1 Plant your feet firmly on the ground with both arms stretched above your head. Close your eyes. Feel a point within yourself (where your center feels located) midway between your head and your feet in the vicinity of your stomach area. Visualize two beams of light (one on side) extending from that center through your arms, to your fingers and from there out into space.

2 Slowly bring your arms down in front of you to shoulder height and hold them outstretched while you keep the image of the light in your mind's eye.

3 As you open your arms sideways, the light follows, stretching forever into space.

4 Bring your arms slowly down to your sides keeping the vision in your mind's eye. The light now reaches deep into the ground. Relax.

Repeat two or three times.

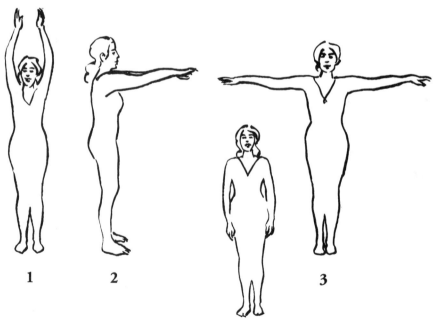

1   2   3

4

5 Stretch your arms back up over your head. Center again. This time the right arm moves slowly forward while the left arm moves backward. Keep thinking of the light stretching into space while you bring both arms down.

6 Do the same movement extending the left arm forward and the right arm backward. Repeat the complete movement two or three times. Relax. Open your eyes.

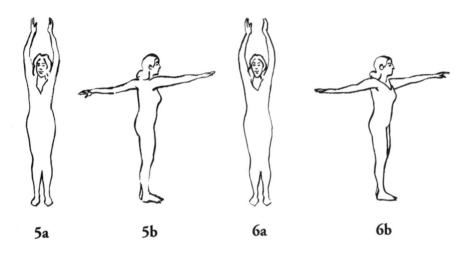

5a   5b   6a   6b

This is your whole living space. When you experience your outer/inner living space, you anchor yourself into yourself. In your inner self, you will always find energy and inspiration.

Practice Lab: The Wheel (daily for one week before going to bed)

I often do this next centering practice in the evening when I feel the need to quiet myself. Lie on the floor, arms placed above and out from your head and legs spread out.

Close your eyes and focus your attention on your heart. Hold your attention there for a few minutes. Open your senses to the feeling inside. Can you feel the pulse of your heart? This is your life pulse. Imagine that your life pulse is moving further down to where your center feels located, midway between your head and your feet. How does it feel? [pause]

Your breath moves in and out. Feel your breath in your center. As you breathe in, you feel the breath moving from your center to your skin, then to the top of your head, to your fingers and toes. Hold your breath gently for a few seconds. When you exhale, your breath flows back to your center. Keep breathing slowly in and out, visualizing the passage of the breath from your center to your periphery and back. [pause]

Imagine yourself contained within a circle whose circumference your fingers and toes can touch. The hub of the wheel is your center. Within is the source of unlimited peace. From this center, every time you breathe in, you fill the circle with energy. As you breathe out, relax and focus on the peace in your heart. [pause]

Continue breathing slowly and quietly. Try to exhale longer than you inhale. Lungs need to be emptied before they can get their fill of fresh air. Soon you feel as though you are in a sphere filled with energy. Stay with it until you feel recharged with new energy.

Practice Lab: Spiritual Centering (daily)

At the end of the day I do my spiritual centering.

1 Sit down comfortably and focus on your heart. Breathe slowly in and out. Imagine (as you did earlier in this Step) the flame of a white candle in the center of your heart. Join the palms of your hands together a few inches from your heart and say to yourself the word "I."

2 In a slow motion, bring your hands together above your head and imagine the white flame expanding toward the top of your head and say the word "am."

3 At the top of your head, your hands part from each other, coming down to your sides until they meet once more, palms joined in front of your abdomen, fingers pointing towards the ground. Imagine the white light moving from your heart all the way to your abdomen and say to yourself, "centering myself."

4 Bring joined hands to your heart, fingers pointing up, saying to yourself, "into myself."

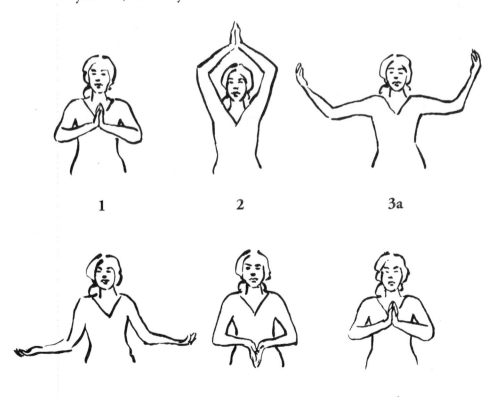

1   2   3a

3b   3c   4

Practice Lab: Quick Centering, Tool 1

Sit or stand, back straight, chest relaxed. Close your eyes. Focus your attention on your center. Breathe slowly in and out for a few minutes. Exhale deeply and slowly as you imagine yourself fully releasing all fatigue and emotional stress. As you inhale deeply, say to yourself, "I am centering myself into myself." Imagine total replenishment of your mental, emotional, spiritual and physical being. Stay with it for a few moments. Slowly open your eyes.

All the Practice Labs can be done several times. Each repetition carries you further along the way. Like practicing scales on the piano, you are working on your inner development, building a new foundation for your celebration of life.

Summary

Centering is a way to achieve wholeness. Your thinking and feeling abilities enlarge your physical potential. When thought, feeling, and senses work in harmony, you are centered.

Journal

Describe your inner space. Describe your center. When you close your eyes and direct your attention to your right hand for several minutes, does it feel warmer? Can you feel how tall you are?

Thought for the Day

Nothing in nature is isolated. Since we are in constant connection with something, we are not separated from the world around us.

Sensuous Awakening Kit, Tool 1: Quick Centering Practice

STEP TWO
Love Thyself

Now that you have learned to center yourself, the next step on your road to self-transformation is to individualize your experience of inner space. You will discover the image of yourself that you carry within and learn to focus on the quality of that image.

Practice Lab: Imaging Self

Close your eyes. What image do you have of yourself? Can you see yourself in your mind's eye? What do you look like facing front? From the back? What does your profile look like? Open your eyes.

Journal: Describe yourself as you appear in your mind's eye.

Role Models

The process of self-perception begins in childhood and continues to develop through puberty and into adulthood. The most powerful influences throughout this process are the role models we choose early in childhood and the way we interpret life's experiences.

The image we find in others and wish to emulate becomes a source of inspiration and security. Your role model might have been your mother or father or even a figure or image who struck your imagination. In my case, it was Anna Pavlova, the Russian ballet dancer who had dazzled the western world at the turn of the century. I was eight when Alexander Volinine, my ballet instructor, introduced me to the legend of Pavlova. His adoration of her was so strong that it seemed to come alive and float on the very air. Her last pair of toe shoes was encased in the hallway leading to his studio. It was there that we children paused to take a deep breath before rushing in to kiss our teacher and to shyly murmur our "Good day!"

Memories of the famous Pavlova lingered throughout the studio for our pleasure and inspiration. My favorite photograph captured her as she sat by the pond of her London house, looking at beautiful swans. A magnificent oil portrait hanging on a studio wall for all to admire brought her to life with all the poetry of her being. Anna Pavlova radiated exquisite grace and taste, and she, with her womanly presence, became my role model at an age when my self-image needed guidance.

Early in my teens, I became quite eager to attract the attention of the opposite sex. School recess was spent in long discussions with my friend Michele regarding which part of our anatomy would likelier attract men—legs, breasts, or a pretty face. We dissected ourselves, assessing our chances in mere pounds of flesh.

It is not uncommon at that age to copy an image, which often acts as a boomerang. The world throws that image back at us. The temptation is to adjust the budding self to what the situation demands, which often creates dilemmas that are compounded by peer pressure and the fear of being left out. The result is that too many young people join the group and behave like sheep in a flock. This, of course, is a danger to healthy development because we must at some point change and propel forward our own strong sense of self. The healthy person integrates a positive image of self which supersedes all the role models, no matter how valuable they have been in the past.

Self-acceptance nurtures a sound self-image. As children, we need love, care and support in our quest for self-acceptance. Unfortunately, many are denied a warm family environment when growing up. And most of us, no matter what our backgrounds, can always use extra encouragement. The following Practice Labs will direct you along the pathway to a strong self-image supported by loving self-acceptance.

Building a Positive Self-Image

What does your appearance communicate to the world? In the same way that your clothes are the outer garment of your personality, your body is the outer garment of your inner Self. It becomes an extension of you.

Go to a full-length mirror and take a good look at yourself. Look at your coloring, the shape of your face, your nose, your eyes. Make mental notes—without judgment—of certain features which are striking to you. Look at your figure. Turn around, so you can observe yourself in movement.

Journal: Describe how you see yourself. Are you the person reflected in your face? In your clothes? In your lifestyle?

Practice Lab: Building Your Image

Before working on your self-image, start with Tool 1, Centering Yourself. Centering prepares you to gather your full energy and prepare for the task at hand. Sit down. Close your eyes. Repeat, "I am centering myself into myself."

Start drawing a mental picture of yourself. Remember your image in the mirror. (Don't worry if the mental image is blurred. It takes practice to work on the mental plane.) Go for the special features you remember. Stay with your image for a little while. Open your eyes.

What did you forget?

Go back to the mirror. Take a second look at yourself. See how your face relates to your torso. How does your torso relate to your arms and legs? Look for relationships. You are now developing a visual sense of flow. You are training your eye to the sensuous discovery of line. Look for curves and the edges. Continue the search for line. How does your head relate to your chest? Look at the angle made by your shoulders. Where does it start? Where does it end? The line moves on down and back up. This is what flow is about. In the same way, everything within—your breathing, circulation, and digestive system—move, change and flow.

Journal: Describe or draw the curves and edges of your face and body. Use the third person. For example: "Her shoulder curves gently..." "Her collarbone is prominent and sharply meets the line of her neck."

Practice Lab: Self-Portrait

Close your eyes. Imagine yourself facing a large canvas. Pick up your paintbrush and begin working on your portrait. First, draw a general outline of yourself and then fill in the details. Refer mentally to your journal notes. Do you remember your proportions? This is your self-portrait. What can you discover about yourself that you did not know before? Write your discoveries in your journal.

Continue adding a line here, a bit of color there, until you are satisfied that you have finished your portrait. Continue the practice of painting your portrait mentally as many times as you can throughout the day until you can do it easily.

Practice Lab: Self-Acceptance

Continue your journey to self-transformation. Go back to the mirror. Take a good look at yourself and observe what it is you do not like. Make three lists in your journal:

List 1: What do you think can be changed easily?

List 2: What can be changed with some work?

List 3: What do you believe cannot be changed?

Self-transformation has to do with change. How can you change something when common sense tells you it is impossible? For example, you want to be tall and lithe, yet you are only five feet two? You cannot change your height, but you can change the feeling you have about it and accept yourself as you are. You are God's creature; you are part of the good which is everywhere in the universe. In the power of good is the power you have to love yourself unconditionally.

Interpretation of Life's Experiences

Let me say something about our past experiences and their influence on our present behavior. (I go into more detail in Step Four.) A part of your mind enables you to tap into both the conscious and unconscious material. However, your mind also contains interpretations of past events which compel you to act in repeated patterns that may severely limit the possibility of any freedom of choice and new behavior. These past interpretations are responsible for reproducing behavior in our daily lives based on experiences that were integrated in the distant past. No longer relevant today, our past continues to deter us from the goal of creating positive change in our lives.

When you clear your mind, you can change this programming. You will release negative emotions which are behind the negative self-image. You will replace these emotions with affirmations that will guide you toward self-acceptance.

Practice Lab: Clearing your Mind, Tool 2 (daily for one week)

Look at the third list in the self-acceptance Practice Lab. Memorize it and then put it aside. Lie down or sit in a comfortable position.

Imagine you are holding a balloon in your hand which needs air. You feel at ease with yourself. Softening your whole body, slowly allow your breath to move in and out three times. On the third exhalation, imagine fear, anger and self-judgment being breathed out into the balloon. [pause]

Continue to fill the balloon. It grows larger and larger. Imagine that all the negative emotions that came to your consciousness are now in the balloon. Place your third list in the balloon. Can you see it inside? Be sure all negative feelings about yourself are out of your system and in the balloon. [pause]

Okay, release the balloon. Let it go. Watch it float away into space and disappear.

Practice Lab: Blanket of Love

Lie down in a comfortable position. Close your eyes.

Focus your attention on your heart. Your breath is quietly moving in and out. Take the time to feel each part of yourself gradually become fully rested. [pause]

Keep your attention on your heart. You are tuning into the wellspring of love in the center of your heart. Be aware of all the love you have ever felt for your loved ones. Include your friends and colleagues. Open yourself to that love pouring in. There is more to come. Allow all the love you have ever felt to build up. Feel it; sense it. It is pouring out of your heart like water overflowing its cup. [pause]

Imagine that each of the millions of cells that constitute your being behaves like a little sponge thirsty for love. See them with your mind's eye and feel how they open themselves to love. All fear, all pain is extinguished. Love is plentiful. It heals and nurtures where it is needed. You feel yourself expanding with deep unlimited love. Divine light is shining through. Love clears and heals all sorrow, all pain, all hate. [pause]

Imagine all the good you have ever done in your life gathering around you like a blanket of love. Imagine all the good thoughts your loved ones, your friends, your colleagues have ever had about you. Imagine these thought forms shining with love and gathering around you. [pause]

Think back in time and space to wherever you have been. Allow happy memories to come to you. In the mental dimension, there is no time-space limitation. See all these loving thoughts gather around you. Feel them, sense them. They form a blanket of love. Gently wrap yourself in this love blanket. [pause]

You deserve all this love. It is yours. Accept it. Linger in it. You have earned it. Affirm: "I fully accept the love I feel. I fully accept it on the mental, emotional, spiritual and physical levels. I fully deserve this love."

Practice Lab: Building Self-Esteem

Post the following affirmation where you can see and repeat it each day:

"The source of my health and beauty flows out of the spirit of love which is the center of my life. It is my privilege to cultivate this spirit with my mental powers."

Summary

Self-acceptance is the support that gives rise to a positive self-image. A healthy self-image includes the whole organism—body, mind, and spirit.

To build a positive self-image, you utilize your mental powers through the techniques of mind-clearing, visualization, and affirmations.

Journal

Glance back over the Practice Labs and describe your self-image. Write about your role models. Is it easy for you to draw a mental image of yourself? What are you learning when you work mentally on your self-portrait? Can you release your negative emotions in the balloon? Can you wrap yourself in the blanket of love?

Thought for the Day

I am learning to see myself through the eyes of love.

Sensuous Awakening Kit, Tool 2: Balloon

STEP THREE
Breathing: The Key to Inner Awakening

As you integrate the practices of this book into your daily life, you will begin to develop an inner ear and eye for subtle changes that are occurring within. Steps One and Two have encouraged you to focus on your newly acquired sense of self. The practice of natural breathing will enhance your awakening further.

Breathing is a function of life. Indeed; it is life itself. The first wail of a newborn infant is the overwhelming proof that he is alive. Breathing is so associated with the living process that the passing of the last breath signifies death.

In Nature, everything is breathing—contracting and expanding— from the smallest cell in the body to the largest mountain on this planet. We humans are part of this universal pulse. If we think of breath as the medium of life, we come to realize that in it we live and have our being.

Breathing happens of its own volition, and should not have to be thought about. It thinks and feels for itself, thank you very much. The problem is that in the past humans have interfered with it, making this beautiful, generous function a victim of our rigidity. We have enslaved it with our mechanistic, self-controlled approach to living. Every time we are afraid, every time the world impinges on us, we hold our breath. Each time a little portion of the joy of life goes, making us the poorer for it.

Breathing is an indicator not only of physical stamina, but of the emotions as well. The English language offers many metaphors that are examples of the emotional and physical interaction of our breathing activity. We say: a breath of spring, breathing space, to take a breather, a breathtaking view, she made me gasp for breath.

Anxiety and fear often originate in the diaphragm, blocking the natural flow of breath. When people speak of tension, they are usually suffering from a physical reaction to psychological factors. A feeling of oppression sets in the chest. The diaphragm becomes rigid. The muscles in the rib cage lose their resilience. The air is no longer expelled properly and breathing becomes shallow.

Breathing is associated with the sympathetic nervous system (involuntary), which is more primitive than the central nervous system (voluntary). For a long time, it was believed there was no correspondence between the two, but the development of biofeedback techniques have proven the contrary. The link is the pneumo-gastric nerve or vagus nerve from the Greek *pneuma* (soul or vital spirit; *vagus* in Latin means vague or meandering). The vagus nerve is the tenth cranial nerve. It links the brain to the sympathetic system. It directly influences the solar plexus—that great network of nerves located directly below the rib cage which supplies the viscera in the abdominal cavity before it ends its meandering in the pelvic girdle.

The ancient philosophers who understood the correspondence between both systems called the solar plexus the "abdominal brain." Through the self-regulatory process of breath function, you can recognize nature's maternal instinct to protect her own.

The breathing cycle of the earth correlates to the seasons. During winter, nature's activity is invisible to the human eye, yet germination is occurring in the seed deep within the soil. At springtime, a bursting activity brings forth the cycle of growth, bud, flower and fruit which continues throughout the summer. At the transition period from summer to fall, the cycle reverses itself. A change is taking place, for what in the past could be seen as outer manifestation will now take place on the inner level. So it is with breathing—in the end is the beginning. You shall see how this relates to your own breathing process.

Practice Lab: Following Your Breath

Lie down. Close your eyes. Take the time to become very quiet in your chest, head and limbs. Become attentive to your bodily sensations, especially the sensation of skin around your face and nose. Feel the contact with the air outside. Become attentive to the in-and-out flow of air through your nostrils.

Can you perceive whether your breathing is:
slow
fast
shallow
deep

Journal: *Describe your breathing.*

Allow your whole self to become quiet. You are perceiving sensory stimuli as the air moves in through your nose... down your throat... towards your chest... and out again. Follow the breath on its way in; follow the breath on its way out. Be adventurous. See if it moves all the way down to your abdomen.

Don't force it. Remember, you cannot make it happen. Keep an attitude of receptivity. As you follow the inner path of your breath, you might become aware of where your path is blocked. When you feel a knot, focus on letting it go. You will discover that, by and by, knots will dissolve!

Deep breathing involves the activity of the abdomen as well as the middle chest. The lower abdomen, called *Tant'ien* by the Chinese, is considered the human reservoir for energy. It is the center from which movement originates. In Zazen (the practice of Zen meditation in Zen Buddhism), the abdomen is the center of power. Breathing into that center (called *hara*) a few inches below the navel creates a sheath of positive vibrations acting on a subliminal level.

I recall the story of a friend of mine who was a Zazen student. While living in New York City, he was cornered by three threatening teenagers. Before they could act, my friend stood in his *hara* position, feeling his ground with mind and breath centered on the abdomen. The youngsters seemed startled. After a moment that seemed like an eternity, the trio turned around and left!

In any ambiguous situation when the outcome seems uncertain, confusion prevails. It is as though Fate gives us a chance to turn the issue to our advantage. My friend, using his *hara* as a self-protective device, became attuned on a subliminal level to a power which neutralized any negative tendencies.

The Outbreath Response

The outbreath response encourages exhalation over inhalation. I never tire of telling my students that unless they empty their lungs first, they cannot take a breath!

With the outbreath response practice, you count your breath slowly which equals the time it takes to say, "one hundred, two hundred, three hundred," and so on.

Practice Lab: The Outbreath Response

The outbreath response operates in three areas of the torso: the abdomen, the middle chest and the upper chest.

Abdomen: Lie on your back, with knees supported by cushions or pillows. Place both hands on your abdomen, just below the navel. Feel your abdomen soften under your hands. Inhale slowly for four counts through the nose, allowing your abdomen to expand as if it was a balloon. Feel the expansion right under your hands. Hold it two counts. Slowly release the abdomen as you exhale (six counts initially, then progress on to eight and then ten). Pause. Do this five times.

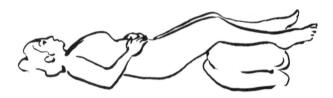

Middle Chest: Same position. Place both hands over the lower part of your rib cage. Allow the breath in through the nose to the count of four, feeling your ribs expand under your hands. Hold for two counts. As you exhale (six to ten counts), bring your hands closer to help push the air out. Pause. Do five times.

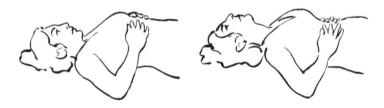

Upper Chest: Same position. Place hands over the sternum (breast-bone) right below the collar bone. As you inhale to the count of four, feel your upper chest open. Hold the breath two counts. As you exhale to the count of six to ten, with both hands press in and down towards the diaphragm. Pause. Do five times.

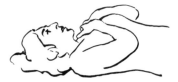 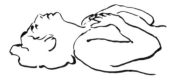

Five Principles

In order to further understand breathing, let's examine five principles. I call them the five functions of breath:

1) Movement
2) Circulation
3) Flow
4) Exchange
5) Transformation

Movement refers to the dual motion of opening and closing. Movement inward, as when air enters the nose, awakens perception of inner space. Outer movement, as when air is released, awakens perception of closing space, much the way a bellows operates. Natural breathing establishes a balance between the dual motions of inhalation and exhalation.

Circulation is the process which carries oxygen to all points in the body through the blood. Through circulation, breath or oxygen is evenly present everywhere. Cyclic in its nature, breath always comes back to its source.

Flow refers to the quality of transition of one cycle into the other. The point of transition calls for a slight pause between inhalation and exhalation, or vice versa. Much is to be discovered in the realization that in the end is already the beginning.

Exchange is when oxygen is passed into the blood and carbon dioxide is released out of the blood. That exchange is the gift of life.

Transformation is renewal. Each breath offers this possibility. The old is forever changed into the new.

Practice Lab: Five Function Awareness

Lie down and close your eyes. Relax your body. Feel the stillness in your limbs and torso reach your head. As you focus on your breathing, meditate on the miracle of life that is represented by the five functions. What image does each function awaken in you?

Journal: Describe the images in your mind's eye when you visualize movement, circulation, flow, exchange and transformation.

Breath Awareness

At a deeper level of consciousness, the air is the vast reservoir of spiritual energy in which we live. The ancients believed breath was sacred. In the Hindu tradition, breath essence is called *prana*, or vital life force. In the practice of Tai Chi, it is called *chi* and the Japanese who practice Zen call it *ki*.

In the Judeo-Christian tradition, breath is the symbol of life. "The Lord God formed man from the dust of the ground and breathed into his nostrils the breath of life. Thus, man became a living creature." (Genesis 7)

And from the Islamic Koran, we find the same symbol. "Your lord said to the angels, 'I am creating man from clay. When I have fashioned him and breathed of My spirit into him, kneel down and prostrate yourself before him.'" (Koran 38:72).

Letting the breath move is what breath awareness is about. It demands your full attention. Mind follows breath. Shunryu Suzuki, Zen Master, said, "The throat is like a swinging door. The air comes in and goes out. It just moves."

The point of this breathing practice is to free the breath. You want to discover what your breath tells you, not impose your will on your breath. The activity of breathing takes place in the whole torso, and indeed your entire being. It affects every cellular fiber; so if I said to you, "Breathe with your big toe," you should be able to feel a sensation in your big toe.

Practice Lab: Breath Awareness, Tool 3

This is a practice that can be done with a friend or alone. Your friend can read it slowly as you respond to the directions. If you choose to do it alone, you can read the directions and perform accordingly, or you can record yourself reading the directions aloud, which will provide another aspect of awareness as you listen to the tone of your own voice.

Lie down, legs propped over a pillow. You will be following your breath with your mind.

Close your eyes. It is as though you let go of your body weight. Feel the impact of the support under you. Shut yourself off from the outside world. Your thoughts become quieter. Center your attention on your breathing. Your chest is very quiet. Breathe in through the nose and allow the breath to open your middle chest, which rises and falls under the breath. . . like the ebb and flow of the sea. [pause]

The breath becomes quieter and deeper. Follow your breath in and out. In... and... out. Each time the breath moves further down. Your abdomen is now rising and falling gently with each breath... like gentle waves rolling in and rolling out. Listen to the sea. Listen to the sea within you. Give your shoulder blades permission to open, inviting the breath to move into that open space. Feel your whole torso rise and fall with the breath. There is nothing for you to do... but be there to receive the breath. The air comes in and out. It just moves... bringing a fresh oxygen supply to the blood, restoring the delicate balance within each cell. [pause]

As the air moves out, it clears the blood of all impurities. Allow your mind to release all negative thought patterns past and present.

As you breathe in, allow positive ideas about yourself... about your work... about the abundance in nature... to flow into your mind and replenish your whole being.

Slowly open your eyes.

Be at peace within.

Summary

The dynamic exchange in the bloodstream between oxygen and carbon dioxide is the gift of life. The outbreath response practice done regularly will help dissolve rigidity in the chest and abdominal area. Breath awareness affects the whole being.

Journal

Can you feel when your breathing becomes shallow? Can you notice change in your breathing when emotions are involved? Have you discovered how deep breathing can dissolve knots? Does meditating on the five functions stimulate a new awareness in your daily activities? What image does each function awaken in you?

Thought for the Day

We share the air with our fellow humans. To be mindful of the breath is to be mindful of the world at large.

Sensuous Awakening Kit Tool 3: Breath Awareness

STEP FOUR
Releasing Tension

Tension is a natural response to a challenge. It is the drive—or sometimes the overdrive—that causes us to act. Without tension, many skills would not exist. Musicians, dancers, athletes and people in business all rely on tension to help them focus on their work. Tension is healthy when it is a part of the process toward the resolution of a situation. However, when tension is present and the situation producing the tension cannot be resolved, then stress sets in.

Stress is being in the middle of conflicting forces. You feel you are being pulled in opposite directions with no resolution in sight. In order to deal with stress, a change needs to occur. The first step is to identify the situation; otherwise you find yourself a victim of whatever is causing the stress. For example, suppose you are crossing the street between traffic lights and a car comes speeding toward you. To meet the challenge, adrenaline is released into your bloodstream and your heart beats faster as you gather every bit of muscle power to run for safety. The emotions that arise activate your "flight or fight" response. This type of stress is easy to identify, and the remedy is simple. You can flatly declare that you will never again take a chance crossing the street! Or you can decide that your built-in "overdrive" is in good condition and carry on. What is important is that you are in charge.

Let's examine physical, mental and emotional stress factors. Some years ago when I started working with music students they would come to me complaining of neck, shoulder or back pains—you name it! The area under stress was different with each instrument. Chronic tension had built up in these musicians because of a lack of basic physical adjustment to the various demands of the instrument. Tension creates a blockage in the muscular structure, preventing the organism from functioning normally. If a change is made in weight distribution, the body will often realign itself and the pain will go away. Being too relaxed is not the solution to physical tension either. Sitting in a slump might provide temporary relief, but in reality we are no better off. If some muscles have totally let go, other groups of muscles have to work twice as hard. A balance between tension and relaxation has to be found in order to create a state of harmony.

When emotions come into play, it is more difficult to define a situation. The "fight or flight" response may not be appropriate. Think back to when you have felt depressed for no apparent reason. You blame the weather or the changing seasons or some other extraneous factor. The depression, in fact, comes from the unconscious. Confusion, anxiety, anger, fear, frustration and sadness are negative emotions that produce stress. They trigger a physiological response recorded as oppression in the chest, pain or cramps in the stomach or abdomen and tightness in the lower back or neck. Sometimes these responses occur for no apparent reason.

Learn to differentiate between stressful situations which can be overcome by identifying them and changing the patterns leading to them, and anxiety, which is produced by undefined emotions.

The Body Reflects Emotional Stress

As a child, I was fascinated by the faces of women. I was attracted to beauty; on the bus ride home from ballet school I made a game of looking for beauty on the faces around me. I noticed that beautifully shaped faces could sometimes be made ugly by long sinuous lines across the forehead or along the cheeks. What's more, I realized that these deep lines were a reflection of the interior selves of the passengers rather than of their surroundings. I wondered why people were unaware of the discrepancy between what was written on their faces and their present situation. I trained myself to become sensitive to subtle changes in my facial expressions and then tried to relate these sensations to my emotions. I discovered that I could live more zestfully if I was aware of my inner and outer feelings simultaneously.

Also, in order not to waste energy, I would observe my habitual movements and catch myself when twisting my body nervously or standing too long on one foot when I had the opportunity to sit. If sitting wasn't possible, I would send a message to both shoulders and back to be perfectly relaxed and not resist, but enjoy the action, whatever it was. You will discover that when mind and body work together, they are a hell of a team! Energy is present, movement flows and the whole self is relaxed.

Practice Lab: Facial Awareness

The following practices have to be done regularly in order for their soothing benefits to be noticeable.

Sit comfortably, hands on lap. How do you feel your face is set? How does it feel around the corners of your eyes? The corners of your mouth? Can you release tension around your mouth and eyes? Try a bigger smile... easy... and let go. Close your eyes gently so the eyelids do not press over the eyes. Open your eyes slowly with just the needed amount of energy... no more... no less. It is up to you to find the right balance.

Relax your forehead. Frown slightly... and let go. Frown again, enough to become aware of your facial motility. Feel the difference between rest and motion, so that your face can be at rest when you are at rest.

During the day, stop periodically and notice how your face is set. Listen to what your face is saying. Take the time to be aware of it while speaking or when preoccupied with your own thoughts. Ask yourself, "Am I conscious of my face right now?" This is what I call self-remembering. Most people perform by rote, as though they were machines.

There are times when you want to be on automatic pilot. For example, when you are playing tennis or skiing or driving you have made the decision to take your self-conscious mind out of the way. You want to feel the groove, to let yourself be on a course and experience the sensation of being one with it. When you stop and return to your self-conscious mind, you heighten your awareness of "being." The practice of self-remembering will help your concentration and is, in fact, a preparation towards greater coordination. This process helps you develop a "sixth sense." The more you do it, the more natural self-remembering will become.

In order to practice self-remembering, you have to distinguish between emotions and feelings. Emotion comes from the word "to move." It is an instinctive feeling. It can also mean that which excites or disturbs. Emotion is a sensation that touches you in such a way that it moves you and often leads to action.

Feeling is a sentiment you experience. It can stay at the level of the mind and of the heart without moving you to action. You might say you are in a state of "being" as opposed to a state of "doing."

Journal: Describe how it feels to relax your face. Now describe how it feels to smile.

Practice Lab: Stress Journal

Stop several times during the day and observe your emotions or feelings. Learn to differentiate between the two.

Journal: Which emotion or feeling relates to this particular physical sensation? And turn the question around: Which physical state relates to this particular feeling or emotion?

Practice Lab: Easing Physical Tension

Tension usually settles in the following areas: 1) behind the eyes; 2) inside the throat and in back of the neck; 3) around the shoulders; 4) in the chest and diaphragm; 5) in the small of the back and 6) in the abdomen.

To soothe the eyes: Make your hands into cups. Place them over your eyes. Keep your eyes open and look into the dark of your palms. Without moving your face, turn your eyes to the left, then to the right, and rest the eyes for about five minutes.

To soothe the throat: Allow the inner membrane of your throat to become quiet, especially the back of the throat, as you keep your mouth closed and breathe quietly through the nose. Concentrate on sensory perception around the tongue and further back where you feel the root of the tongue is. Shift your attention to the lower jaw and relax it until your lower lip gently moves open. Rest.

To relax the back of the neck: During exhalation, allow your chin to fall onto your chest with your head bent down. Take a deep breath in, followed by a deep breath out. On the next inhalation, slowly bring your head up. As you exhale, move your head to the right, then to the left and center. Rest.

To relax the chest and diaphragm: Lie on your back with knees supported by cushions. Place both hands over the lower part of your rib cage. Allow the breath in through your nose to the count of four, feeling your ribs expand under your hands. Hold for two counts. As you exhale (6 to 10 counts), bring your hands closer together to help push the air out. Pause. Do five times.

To relax the small of the back: Lie down. Wrap your arms around your knees and bring them as close as possible to your chest. Exhale. When you are ready to inhale, release the pressure. Do it a few times until your back feels fully stretched.

To relax the stomach and abdomen: Lie on your back with knees supported by cushions. Place your hands on your abdomen, directly below the navel. Feel your abdomen soften under your hands. Inhale slowly for four counts through the nose, allowing your abdomen to expand as though it were a balloon. Hold for four counts. Slowly release the abdomen as you exhale six to eight counts. Pause. Do five times.

Mental Stress

In his book, *The Dragons of Eden,* Carl Sagan mentions Paul McLean's comparison of the human brain to three interconnected biological computers. It is generally accepted today that the intrauterine development of the human fetus can be equated with the three stages of evolution. The fetus at first resembles a fish, then a mammal and finally a human. McLean states that the most ancient brain is comprised of the spinal cord, hind brain and mid-brain—called the R complex—which we share with reptiles. It regulates reproduction and self-preservation, or instinct.

Our "mammal" brain, called the limbic brain, surrounds the R complex. It includes the pituitary gland and other glands which strongly influence the endocrine system. It came later and its function is to generate the strong emotions regulated by genetic input, or by one's own nature.

The neo-cortex is a more recent evolutionary development and is the site of human cognitive functions. We share this development with whales and dolphins. Although the neo-cortex accounts for 85% of brain mass, humans revert to their more primitive brain when instinctive and emotional concerns arise.

What does all this have to do with mental stress? We know that the "fight or flight" response relates back to when people had to fight daily for their lives. We could, according to McLean's theory, assume that the R complex is responsible for "fight-or-flight" behavior and the limbic brain for moods unrelated to objective reality.

The mind is divided into conscious and unconscious material, and the personality is formed by our ability to process both. Most people unconsciously resist change and so the personality sets limits (through our habits) as we grow older. We cling to the familiar where we feel safe, much the way a child clings to its mother, yet life continuously demands that we grow and change.

When the opportunity to advance in consciousness comes up there is a tremendous demand for adjustment to the new situation and often our whole belief system feels threatened. The unconscious resists the new, and people become strongly attached to their neuroses, which causes chronic anxiety and stress. Bring them to light, and healing takes place.

In the summer of 1987 I found myself exposed financially for the first time in my life. My husband and I had a mortgage on the apartment of our dreams in Virginia. We decided to pay it off by buying and then selling our rent-controlled Manhattan apartment (which had just turned co-op). Feeling very optimistic about the outcome, we took a one-year lease on a large studio in the city. Now we were committed to *two* mortgages, *two* monthly maintenance charges, and a rental fee.

Then came Black Monday, the Wall Street crash of 1987. I felt like a ship out to sea when the storm hits. Why was I not quietly anchored in the harbor waiting for the gale to pass? All my hidden fears and self-doubts came crawling out to call me by all kinds of names. My self-judging thoughts had a field day.

Well, how long can you torture yourself? I knew I must change my attitude and I had better do it fast! My intuition told me that the crisis offered a chance to test my trust in life. If indeed I believed, as I thought I did, that prosperity and harmony are inherent qualities in every life situation, I had to get to work. Every morning upon waking and every night before going to bed, I affirmed in the silence of my heart that a perfect situation, for the good of all concerned, was in the making. Within a week our studio was rented.

For the next six months I had plenty of time to reinforce my new outlook on life. It was so tempting to go back to the old fears. I had to reaffirm daily my trust in the good of life. At the same time I actively took responsibility for resolving the impact of this crisis on our finances. It paid back a hundred fold. During this time of worldwide financial insecurity, the real estate market was extremely soft. Logically, the value of our apartment in Manhattan should have plunged. However, through consistent, focused work we were able to attract three buyers. We sold it for precisely the money we needed to realize our dream. In addition, many small miracles occured to bring us money we had not counted on. Since then I have daily reasons to believe my life is prosperous. Even when outer appearances are bleak, one's destiny can unfold harmoniously. I learned that a combination of positive affirmation (trust) and hard work bring us everything we need in life.

Looking at a situation or problem head-on adds a new perspective to one's life which leads to transformation. This perspective is a source of well-being. When you succumb to the pull of negative emotions you separate yourself from your source of well-being, where all is harmony.

Anger, sadness and fear—when unconsciously acted out—prevent access to new insights.

Practice Lab: Clearing Process, Tool 4

The liver is said to be the seat of anger. Lie down, close your eyes. Center yourself, breathing quietly. Focus your attention on your right side, directly below the rib cage where the liver is located. On each inbreath, imagine every liver cell being renewed. On each outbreath, imagine toxins being released. In your center, or inner sanctum, you are saying to yourself, "I give each cell in my liver permission to be clear of anger."

The spleen is said to be the center of sadness. Lie down, close your eyes. Center yourself by breathing quietly. Focus your attention toward your left side, below your rib cage where the spleen is located. On each inbreath, imagine each cell being restored to health. On each outbreath, imagine toxins leaving your spleen. In your inner sanctum, you are saying, "I give each cell in my spleen permission to clear all the sadness that has ever been in my past."

The stomach is said to be the seat of fear. Lie down, close your eyes. Center yourself, breathing quietly. Focus your attention on your lower chest where your solar plexus is located. (The solar plexus is a great network of nerves and ganglia situated behind your stomach and in front of the diaphragm.) You are very quiet and relaxed. As you breathe deeply, feel your lower chest and abdomen open on each inbreath. As you exhale, release your lower chest and abdomen. How relaxed are you in your stomach area? How tense? Do you know what your stomach looks like? If not, find an anatomy book. I strongly suggest that you get to know your stomach and how it reacts to your daily activities. Can you make a connection between the image of your stomach and what it feels like?

On each outbreath, imagine bubbles of fear being released out of the stomach and replaced on the inbreath by new cells. Imagine your genetic coding no longer affected by negative tendencies, but reflecting instead the original blueprint of peace, love and harmony. You are saying to yourself, "I give each cell in my stomach permission to be clear of fear."

Journal: Write a conversation between your higher self and each of your internal organs, in which you state the permissions described above, and write the reply that comes to your imagination.

Practice Lab: Daily Affirmation

This affirmation will harmonize you physically, mentally and spiritually. With this new state of mind, you will acquire more resilience to deal with stress.

Sit on the edge of a chair with your back straight, feet apart and firmly on the ground, arms along your sides.

First, gently drop your head onto your chest so its weight pulls on your neck and shoulders. Keep lowering your head until your entire torso is resting on your lap with your head fully down, hanging between your knees. Pay attention to your breathing. As you exhale, you are flushing out negative thoughts. As you breathe in, visualize new, fresh positive thoughts rushing into your bloodstream. Slowly roll up your spine and say to yourself, "I am totally renewed in mind, body and spirit."

Practice Lab: Relaxation into Oneness

The perfect time to cultivate a state of oneness is at the end of the day when you lie down, before falling asleep.

Lie comfortably and close your eyes.

Become aware of your breathing. Breathe in through your nose, giving yourself time to feel the breath go all the way to your abdomen. On each breath, your abdomen rises and falls evenly... there is nothing for you to do, nothing at all. [pause]

Release the tension in your feet [pause]... in your ankles [pause]... and in your knees. Let the muscles in your legs soften. [pause]

A lovely feeling of relaxation enters your hands, your arms and your trunk [pause]... now it reaches your shoulders [pause]... your throat and your head [pause].

You feel as if you are floating. Experience the sensation of stillness in your feet and hands. From your extremities it goes upward along your arms and your legs [pause]... stillness moves higher up along your spine and moves up everywhere... stillness is all over you. [pause]

Focus on your heart... in your heart, experience the feeling of tranquillity. Tranquillity is moving deeper and deeper into the layers of your heart. It feels as though ripples of tranquillity are entering the heart of every cell in your body. [pause]

Focus your attention inside your head. In your mind center, invite the feeling of peace... peace is entering every thought you hold in your mind... layer upon layer of mental activity is impregnated with peace [pause]... it is as though peace were permeating your essence, blending with tranquillity and stillness into one essence, the source of your being.

Summary

Stress is the result of unresolved mental or physical tension. When you identify the source of tension you can make conscious changes that will eliminate the stressful situation.

Affirmation and self-induced relaxation is a therapeutic way to dissolve deep-seated stress. Daily practice in self-awareness will free you from old behavior patterns.

Thought for the Day

Your face is the mirror of your thoughts.

Journal

Describe how you feel when you are tense. Describe how you feel when you are stressed. Write about the difference between emotions and feelings, giving examples from your own life. Describe how your face is set right now. Do you resist change? If so, write about your resistance. Are you regularly using your tools from Steps One, Two and Three? Are you noticing a change in your breathing habits?

Sensuous Awakening Kit, Tool 4: Clearing Process

STEP FIVE
Creating Balance Through Polarity

In ancient times, knowledge was transmitted orally, a method that kept traditions alive from generation to generation. These stories were filled with abstract concepts about God and creation and included lessons in behavior as well. The poetic quality of the parables stimulated the imagination and the intuition of the listener. Our ancestors treated nature with respect. They recognized its sacred character and worshipped the principles that govern it.

Polarity, or the manifestation of two opposite principles, one negative and one positive, is one of the themes that emerges from ancient literature. The law of polarity is also contained in Oriental cosmology, where the world is seen as the interaction of two complementary opposites—Yin and Yang. In this belief system, the original undifferentiated Absolute divided itself into two aspects. Yin, the female principle, has the attributes of yielding and receiving and is moist. Its energy is also expansive in Nature. Yang connotes firmness, arising and is dry. Yang energy moves toward a center. The basic precept of this philosophy is that all existence is one and that life is the result of the harmony that exists between these two poles.

Many mystics over the centuries had intuitively perceived some form of energy basic to body maintenance which had no physical form. Then in the eighteenth century, Luigi Galvani and Count Alessandro Volta of Italy discovered the principle of electricity. This force, until then hidden in Nature and unknown to sense observation, is the result of two complementary types, negative and positive. Our western world was transformed when this revolutionary idea was discovered. Unfortunately, in our culture only materialistic benefits were drawn from it. In terms of Chinese philosophy, we neglected the spiritual aspect of its application. We impoverished our culture of what the German mystic Rudolph Steiner called "the mysterious power which dwells in the soul of Nature, deeply hidden like the electrical force."

The Chinese system of medicine is based on the balance of the opposites. Practitioners see the human body as a microcosm of the universe, regulated by the same principles that govern the interaction of positive and negative forces. They hypothesized that *chi* energy, or the vital life force, has both negative and positive aspects. When the imbalance occurs between the two, vital centers become clogged and exhaustion sets in, often followed by physical and mental illness. The system is cleared when balance is reinstated. Vitality is again high; and health, appearance and joy of life are at their maximum.

The same polarity principles apply in our daily lives as well. When we look around us, we find that each phenomenon is dual in nature. Day is followed by night, summer by winter, our fortunes go up or down, we can go right or left. A positive and a negative principle is constantly operating. What lies midway between these two poles is change, as one phenomenon moves into its opposite. We will examine two aspects of polarity: the aspect of change that leads to transformation, as one phenomenon is transformed into its opposite, and the aspect of balance which is so beautifully expressed in the words of T. S. Elliot:

> *"At the still point of the turning world. Neither flesh nor fleshless;*
> *Neither from nor towards; at the still point, there the dance is,*
> *But neither arrest nor movement. And do not call it fixity,*
> *Where past and future are gathered."—(Four Quartets)*

The two contrasting forces that affect you most are gravity, which keeps your feet on the ground, and *chi* energy, which is a measure of your vitality. When the two combine, you can perceive the sensuous quality of your life.

My understanding of the dynamics of gravity came with my discovery of Flamenco dancing. In the 1960s, I went to live in Madrid. At the time I was married to a screenwriter and outstanding movies were being made in Spain. My life in Madrid offered many interesting opportunities, and I settled into some of the most enriching years of my life.

I immediately felt at home with the warmth and directness of the Spanish people. There was an abundance of energy everywhere, particularly in the way people expressed themselves with their hands and eyes in order to emphasize the meaning of their words. I loved their language and came to speak it fluently. I loved their music, so I took up guitar. But most of all, I loved Flamenco dancing and I decided to study it seriously. Every day I worked with the famous Rosario (of the dance team Rosario and Antonio), who had recently retired, learning intricate combinations of footsteps and arm movements that followed very specific patterns. Then I would spend the rest of the day at the Dance Academy with La Quica, where I practiced my steps.

I was fascinated by the long and sinuous torsos of the professional dancers, the graceful carriage of their heads and the supple movements of their wrists and hands. The women were proud of their busts and of their femininity. They radiated a natural sensuality without affectation.

The energy released by their footwork alternated with the graceful positioning of their bodies. At times their bodies were completely still, as though the dancers were gathering the energy which was to be poured into the next step seconds later. The Spanish dancer is aware of the floor when performing. Her center of gravity, low in the pelvic structure, is being centered towards the earth—the reverse of the ballet dancer who pulls that center up, and must fight gravity in order to achieve elevation.

I began to understand the importance of polarity. The connection with the earth gives one energy and, like the ballet dancer, you can let it flow up to reach towards heaven! You can be aware of your connection with the ground while sitting, standing or lying; simultaneously you can be alive and present in your tissues and feel your body weight distributed. You radiate energy. What a discovery! It is so simple. All you have to do is give Mother Earth her due!

Working with Polarity and Vital Life Force

Practice Lab: Gravity-Dive to the Earth

Movement, too, has a dual nature. What contracts also expands. Everything that is alive, down to the simplest form of life, the amoeba, is in constant motion. Imagine the millions of cells in your system pulsating with life energy, contracting and expanding as each one divides into a sister cell, causing life to go on.

Stand up, feet firmly grounded, arms along your sides. Drop your chin onto your chest. Relax your shoulders and let your knees unlock. Allow the full weight of your head to bear down so it pulls on your neck and shoulders. The head leads the way as it pulls you down, with the spine following, vertebra by vertebra. You feel you are being pulled by the sheer force of gravity until you are doubled in from the waist down, firmly supported by your legs. Enjoy the sense of letting go. Slowly roll up your spine, vertebra by vertebra as you gently straighten your knees, making sure your legs are firmly supporting you. After your shoulders and neck are up, bring your head up.

Adjust your breathing to this practice. As you go down, you will find it easier to start by exhaling deeply. As you start the roll up, you will find that breathing in deeply is helpful. Practice several times a day.

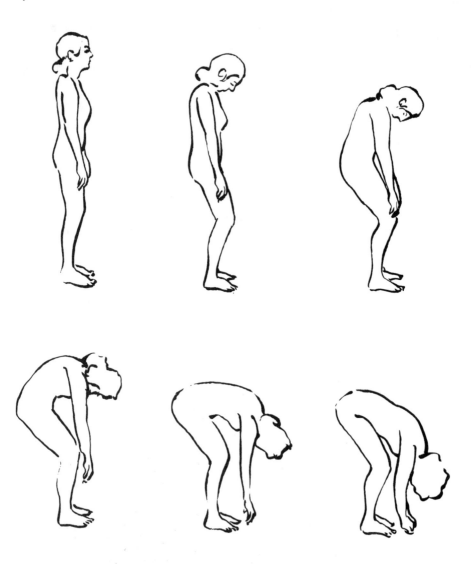

Practice Lab: Vital Life Force—Reaching to the Heavens

1 Stand up. Plant your feet firmly on the ground. Raise both arms above your head. Stretch your right arm as high as you can. Relax.

2 Stretch your left arm as high as you can. Relax.

3 Stand on tiptoes. Simultaneously, reach up with both arms as high as you can. Hold your balance as long as you can. Relax. Do two or three times in a row.

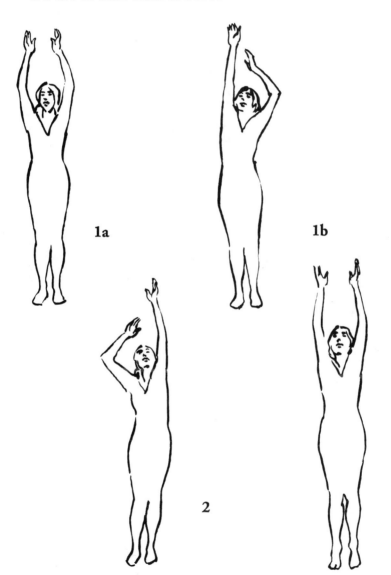

1a

1b

2

3

Practice Lab: Polarity Walk—Dual Aspect of Balance

If possible, walk on bare ground. As you begin walking, make sure your shoulders and chest are relaxed, and your spine erect. Gradually, become aware of the ground under your feet. A sensuous feeling enters your feet. It is as though you are absorbing earth energy through your feet. Allow that energy to move up like sap along your legs as you walk, sensing the ground. The energy courses on up the spine, helping you to stand straighter. Stop and raise your arms and stand on tiptoe, as high as you can.

Continue walking on tiptoe with your arms up. Your point of gravity has shifted from your abdomen to a position midway between your fingers and your toes. Can you feel where it is? Can you stretch your arms higher as you walk? Think of yourself pushing against the ground in order to go higher. Do you feel like you could take off and fly?

Now it is time to enter the transition where one movement converts to its opposite. As you continue moving forward, your heels come down, then gradually bring your shoulders, arms and elbows down. Keep walking as you unlock your knees and your arms slide down your sides. Cave your shoulders in and pull your chin down. It is as though the spine has let go, succumbing to the pull of the earth. Relax your back and allow your breath to adjust to the change. Your point of gravity has shifted further down your trunk.

Walk through the full sequence four or five times and rest. Focus on transition. Be aware of the environment, the air you breathe, the ground you walk on and the space you travel through.

Know that you are part of everything that touches your senses and everything is part of your experience. You are an open system receiving and giving energy.

Increasing Your Energy

You take vital energy from the elements; that is, the energy of the universe is converted into individual energy. Like plants, we are revived by exposure to light and water. Like animals, we are revitalized by the air we breathe and the food we eat. When fresh air containing chi is inhaled, it invigorates and heals the body. The surplus is stored in the solar plexus, thus creating a reserve tank. As human beings, we are stimulated by the thoughts we have and the impressions we receive. You improve the quality of energy when you are fully present in the moment, when your heart is in it. And when fully at one with your creative mind, you become whole.

Practice Lab: Foot Stomping

Stand up in a relaxed position on a thick rug if possible, as it will reduce the noise and offer additional support. With sensitivity, not with strength, allow one foot to stamp on the floor, then the other. You are making contact with the floor, not hitting it. Your knees are flexed, your back straight. Take time to feel the impact each time your foot touches the floor. Keep going faster and faster as your steps become smaller and smaller. It is as though you are shaking all over. Do five minutes.

Preserving Energy

You can save energy by learning to use only what is necessary and no more. This is achieved by being fully in the moment. Incredible amounts of energy are wasted by activities such as idle chit-chat or worry and anxiety.

Practice Lab: Isolations

Isolation is the practice of moving one part of the body without interfering with the rest. You can isolate any part. For example, you can close your right eye without moving the left. Try. Practice eye isolation until you feel comfortable with it. Try to use just enough energy to close your eyes without tensing the forehead.

Shoulder Isolation: Lie on your back on the floor. Move your right shoulder joint forward a few inches away from the floor, hold it for two counts, let it go back to the floor. Make sure everything else is perfectly still. Do it four times, then do the left shoulder.

Hip Isolation: Lie on your back on the floor. Move your right hip up a few inches off the floor, hold it two counts, let it go. Do it four times, then turn to the left hip. This exercise represents quite a challenge as it is not easy to mobilize the group of muscles directly connected with your hip without involving the thigh. Don't get discouraged. Try and you will succeed!

Journal: Describe how it feels to do these exercises.

Practice Lab: Energy Flow

1 Sit down comfortably, back straight, feet grounded. Your left
   hand rests turned out on your left thigh while your right hand is
   turned palm down on your right thigh. Your left hand
   corresponds to your Yin side (negative, feminine, receiving).
   Your right hand is your Yang side (positive, masculine, giving).
   Breathe evenly and peacefully, quieting your thoughts. Tune
   your mind to the inner experience of being centered. After a
   few minutes, turn your attention to your left hand. Can you
   feel the energy being pulled in? (Imagine a little vacuum
   cleaner.) Turn your attention to your right hand as it contacts
   your right thigh. Can you feel the energy build up through your
   being? Can you feel it flow through and through?

2 After a while, turn your left palm down on your left thigh and
   close your eyes. Stay quiet. The energy is now self-contained.
   Experience the flow for as long as it feels necessary after you have
   closed your eyes.

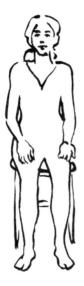 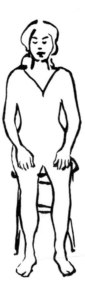

Journal: *Describe the difference of feeling between having your palm up
and your palm down in this exercise.*

Tuning to Higher Energies

Can we tune to finer or higher energies? According to India's sacred texts, you have seven centers or *chakras* in your being which harbor divine energy. These centers are distributed along the spine. Each acts as a focus of consciousness. Each center corresponds to a spiritual, mental, emotional and physical reality. Like notes on a scale, they resonate to a lower or higher pitch of frequency according to their position on the spine and to the individual's state of inner development.

These centers of consciousness are channels of subtle energies that enable one to discover his or her special attunement with the universe. The first three *chakras*, located in the lower part of your trunk, relate to lower nature and are influenced by earth energy; the last four *chakras*, located in the upper portion of your being, relate to your higher nature.

The first, or root *chakra*, is located at the base of the spine. It relates to the earth energy and to the functions of assimilation and elimination.

The second, or navel *chakra*, is located at the first lumbar vertebra about one inch below the navel. It relates to the activity of the sexual glands and presides over the function of childbearing.

The third, or spleen *chakra*, is located at the eighth dorsal vertebra and relates to the solar plexus. It regulates hepatic and splenic activities as well as the sympathetic nervous system. It serves as a point of balance and transformation of the grosser into the more subtle energies.

The fourth, or heart *chakra*, is located at the seventh cervical vertebra. It relates to coronary and pyloric activity as well as to the thymus gland. It is the seat of love energy.

The fifth, or throat *chakra*, is located at the third cervical vertebra. It relates to the thyroid gland and influences metabolic activity. It is the center of self-empowerment and self-expression.

The sixth, brow *chakra* or third eye, is located at the first cervical vertebra. It relates to the pineal and pituitary glands. Once developed, the sixth *chakra* becomes a center of heightened consciousness and extrasensory perception.

The seventh, or crown *chakra*, is at the top of the head and relates to pure consciousness, the seat of the higher self and oneness with God.

In the same way that a musical instrument has to be tuned in order to play harmoniously, *chakra* centers have to be kept in a state of proper balance. The following Practice Labs are two ways of keeping them in tune.

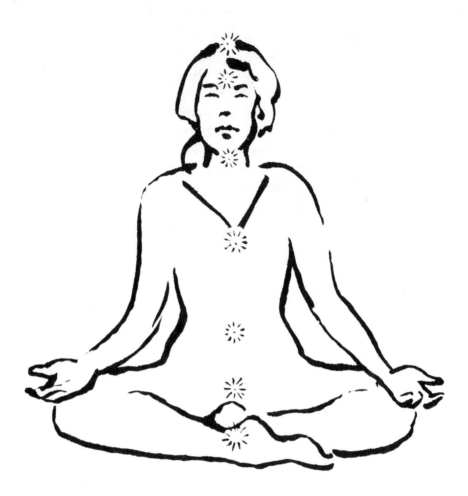

Practice Lab: Chakra Meditation

Sit comfortably keeping your back straight and your hands on your lap. Close your eyes. Imagine a ball of divine light above the crown of your head. The light vibrates perfect love, harmony and life. Focus on its radiance and visualize the light entering your crown, instantly illuminating the inside of your head. The light moves down and suffuses your throat area. Beams of light move down your spine, flooding your chest, diaphragm, and abdomen with divine light. It flows down your legs, radiating its light into the earth. Your whole being pulsates with vibrant, loving, life-giving energy. Take plenty of time to experience this.

Journal: Describe your experience of this exercise.

Practice Lab: Chakra Attunement, Tool 5

Stand in a relaxed position and do Tool 1, Quick Centering. Place your left hand a few inches away from the base of your spine (palm turned in) where your first *chakra* is located. Place your right hand in front of your abdomen, holding it a few inches away. Center your breathing into your abdomen. Hold the position for 15 seconds. Bring both hands in the same position to your navel *chakra*. Hold it for 15 seconds. Move your hands in the same spatial ratio over each chakra. In order to reach the heart *chakra* with your left hand, reach over your left shoulder. When you are about to reach the crown *chakra* (seventh) only your right hand moves to the crown of the head. Your left hand stays in the back of the brow *chakra*. Hold this position for 15 seconds. Keeping your right hand over your crown *chakra*, slowly lower your left hand to your throat *chakra* for a few seconds. Slowly lower your right hand to meet your left, then gently brush the energy over your shoulders and down your back towards the ground. Relax.

Summary

You are an open system, receiving and radiating energy. You function within the polarity of a gravitational field and the vital energy, or *chi*, which animates all things.

From the top of your head to the base of your spine are seven centers of consciousness which you can develop through the practice of meditation and special attunement.

Thought for the Day

As a child of both Heaven and Earth, you need to rediscover your natural inheritance.

Journal

Write about your bodily and emotional sensations when you are depleted. Write about how it feels when you are charged up. Can you discover the transition point between these two states and consciously experience balance? Can you be fully present in the moment, whether you are brushing your teeth or working at a computer? Has your breathing changed since you began your self-transformation? Is your life more stress-free?

Sensuous Awakening Kit, Tool 5: Chakra Attunement

STEP SIX
Tuning Up

On your journey of transformation you discovered your center and reinforced your self-image. You have awakened to new breathing possibilities, increased your ability to deal with stress and expanded your awareness of the laws of polarity. Now you have arrived at the edge where the inner becomes the outer; the form reflects the idea. In this Step I will begin leading you into the physical realm of your transformation. With discipline—and with a realistic goal in mind—you will obtain wonderful results.

Your physical transformation stretches over the next three Steps and will require five weeks to be completed. You will then continue your daily maintenance program (the Dance) which will take no more than seven minutes a day. In the first week (Tune-up: this Step) you warm up every day building up your strength and limbering your joints with Practice Labs. The next three weeks are devoted daily to muscle tone (Workout: Step Seven).

In the fifth week (Step Eight) you start practicing the sequence of the Dance movements, warming up first with your Tune-up program. In the sixth week, you are ready to do the Dance. The Dance becomes your only daily maintenance program; however, it is advisable to do a thorough session combining the Tune-up and the Workout once a week.

Your body contains millions of receptors which feed data about your inner and outer state of being to the central nervous system. These receptors are constantly monitoring muscle tension, body temperature, pain and sensory impressions. Sensory impressions normally refer to outside stimuli but can also include inner perception and were emphasized, as you will recall, in the centering process you learned in Step One.

When you gather your energy in order to start on a task, you are tuning in to the environment as well as to the energy inside you. Tuning up—the practice of activating muscles gradually and loosening joints and tendons at the same time—prevents stiffness and unnecessary accidents.

Years ago, with the aid of a chiropractor and my own self-created movement practices, I overcame a chronic problem which had threatened to limit my activities. (Not only was my problem solved, but it turned out to be a blessing in disguise because it opened the door to my current profession.) I created a program of limbering the spine. I chose movements which could stretch each vertebra equally in order to realign my spine along the head/neck/back axis. I rediscovered my joints and started to give them the attention they deserve.

A joint or articulation is the connecting medium between bones. Ligaments are the tough, fibrous tissues which bind bones together. If you could take a peek inside your joints, you would discover a lining called the synovial membrane that secretes a fluid that lubricates the joint. Special attention in a tune-up assures the optimum level of lubrication.

Let's do a practical experiment. Use the following symbols:

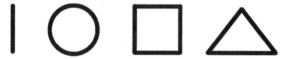

Copy the above shapes onto a piece of paper in an arrangement that resembles the human body. Make a vertical line in the center of the paper to represent the spine. Place the circle at the top. Come down an inch below the circle and draw a square for the rib cage. Two more lines extending from the top corners of the square will serve as arms. A reversed triangle creates the pelvic structure or lower torso and two more vertical lines extending down from the base of the upside-down triangle form the legs.

What do you see at first glance? You see single units: the head, neck and torso. And you see pairs: arms and hands, legs and feet. What connects pairs to single units are two strong hinges (the shoulders and hips) and the neck. Single units need to be centered around your central axis (your spine) of which your neck is a part. Your neck is formed by seven cervical vertebrae, the first of which is called Atlas. In mythology, Atlas is the Titan who carries earth on his back. Atlas, your first of seven vertebrae, holds your head in balanced motions with your neck and spine. Twelve thoracic, five lumbar, your sacrum and coccyx are the other vertebrae that form your spine.

Your head and trunk, or single units, contain organs which contribute to your being. The head is unique in that it harbors the conscious center, the brain, which in turn depends totally on the cardiovascular and digestive systems for its life activity. Your heart and digestive system can function without your brain, but your brain cannot function without them. Think about it!

The trunk contains the heart center and breathing center in the upper part, the torso and the digestive system in the lower part or pelvic area. The experience of self as a living organism is the result of a dynamic relationship between being and doing. It is an alliance between mobility and support, functions that are both autonomous and interdependent.

Arms and legs, on the other hand, signify activity, mobility and freedom. The arms and hands have the most mobility while the legs and feet have the important function of supporting your whole weight. A builder knows by experience that unless the foundations of his high-rise are sound, he will not have a secure building. Similarly, we shall start working on the body foundation. These observations will help when you organize your Tune-up or Warmup program.

Practice Lab: Preparation

Stand in a relaxed position. As you stand, can you feel whether your right side is equally balanced with your left side? Now prepare your alignment with the earth by doing a mini-pendulum.

Mini-pendulum sideways: Feet together, shift your weight to your right side, then to your left and back to center. Close your eyes for a few seconds to appreciate in your inner self the change in your alignment.

Mini-pendulum forward and back: Feet together, shift your weight forward, then slowly backward and back to center. Close your eyes and evaluate your new position.

This preparation should take about 15 seconds and can be applied any time your Tune-up and Workout routines require a standing position. Aligning yourself with the earth, you develop a spatial relationship with your center of gravity.

TUNE-UP (first week, 10 minutes daily)

The first session may take up to 30 minutes as you read instructions and learn the movements.

Practice Lab: Your Support System

Your feet make constant adjustments with the ground while they support your weight. The position of your whole structure depends on their flexibility.

Stand behind a chair (high-backed if possible), feet parallel, a comfortable distance apart. Rest the fingertips of your hands on top of the chair.

1 Raise your heels and stand up on your toes as high as you can. Hold five seconds.
2 As you bring your heels down, shift your weight back on your heels and raise your toes upward. Hold five seconds.
   Do ten times.

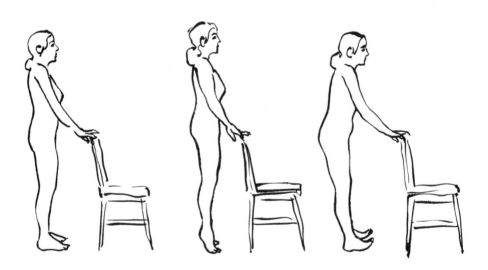

1   2

3 With feet flat on the floor, roll slowly towards the outer edges so the inner soles lift up. Hold five seconds.
4 Press the inner soles down so the outer soles come up. Hold five seconds. Do ten times.
5 Pull in your toes as if you wanted to grab something. Hold five seconds.
6 Stretch toes wide apart. Hold five seconds.
   Do five times.

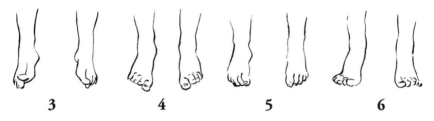

3   4   5   6

Practice Lab: Knee Bend

Stand, feet together, behind a chair. Rest your fingertips on top of the chair.

1 Bring your right knee up as high as you can. Keep your back straight. Hold for five seconds. Bring your right foot down.
2 Bring your left knee up as high as you can. Hold for five seconds. Bring your left foot down.
   Do ten times.

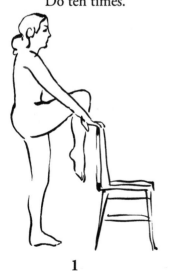 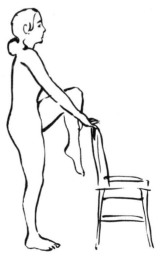

1   2

Practice Lab: Pelvic Tilt

Stand, feet together, behind a chair. Rest your fingertips on top of the chair.

1 Tilt your pelvis forward, contracting your abdomen in and tightening your buttocks together. Feel your lower spine lengthen. Hold five seconds.
2 Relax your back completely.
   Do six times.

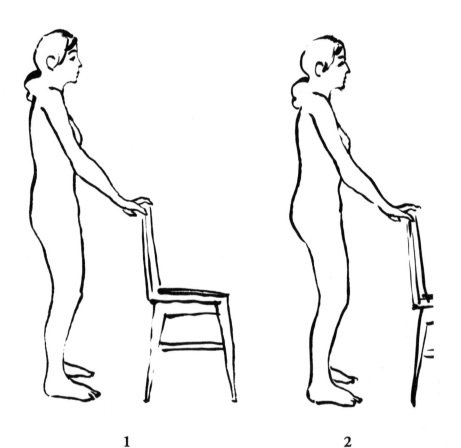

1   2

Practice Lab: Spinal Alignment

Your spine is made up of 24 vertebrae. It supports the head and the back, and its position determines the suppleness of your gait and your general well being.

Stand up, feet slightly apart, knees relaxed. Drop your chin and head down onto your chest, then your shoulders, your arms and so on. Eventually, your torso is doubled from the waist down. Relax for a few seconds. Take a deep breath in, then exhale. Keep your knees relaxed. Inhale, rolling your spine up slowly, making sure your shoulders come up first, then your neck and finally your head. Do four times.

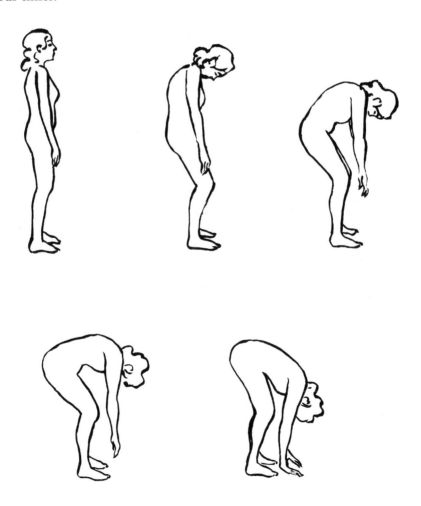

Practice Lab: Spatial Orientation

You are defined by your place on the physical level as well as by your position in your consciousness. Do you remember working with your living space in Step One? Here you are working with your four cardinal points. If you decide your head is the North Pole, your feet become the South Pole, your right hand is West and your left hand is East.

Lie down. Close your eyes. Make some adjustments along your north/south axis until it feels perfectly straight. Open your eyes.

Practice Lab: Back Stretch

1 Lie on your back, both legs bent over your chest, your arms encircling your knees.
2 Bring your knees closer and closer to your chest. Push your shoulders back to the floor, so your back is as flat as possible. Hold for the duration of a full exhalation.
3 Relax your shoulders, place your hands flat over your kneecaps and hold tightly. Shift the weight of your knees forward until your arms are stretched to their fullest and both shoulders are forward. Keep your head on the floor. Hold for the duration of a full inbreath. Relax.
Do four times.

1   2   3

Practice Lab: Knee Crossover

1 Lie on your back with both knees bent and your feet on the floor. Extend your arms in a T position.
2 Bring your right knee over your chest.
3 Cross your knee over the line of your spine toward your left side until both knees fall as close to the ground as possible on your left. Keep your hands touching the floor as your right shoulder gently lifts. Turn your head in the opposite direction and hold four counts.

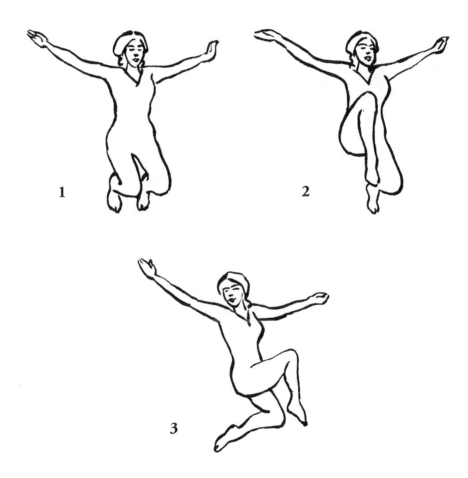

4 Bring your right knee back over your chest and your head back
   to center. Gently lower your right foot to the ground.
     Repeat 2 through 4, this time bringing the left knee to the right.
Do twice each side.

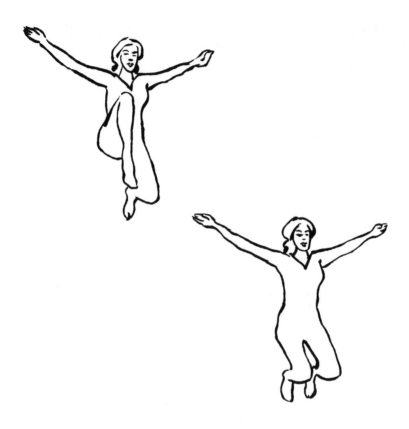

Practice Lab: Head to Knee Stretch

1 Lie on your back, knees bent over your chest, feet off the floor, hands behind your head with elbows flat on the floor. Breathe in deeply.

2 When you are ready to breathe out, bring your head up to meet your knees with elbows forward into a tuck. Maintain the "egg" position as long as you are exhaling. As you inhale, bring your elbows and your head back to the floor.

Do four times.

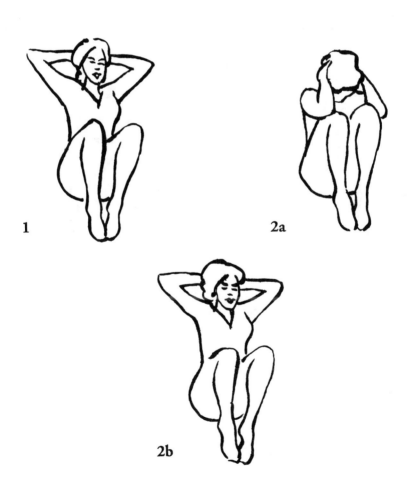

1   2a

2b

Practice Lab: Shoulders, Head and Neck

Imagine for a moment that your shoulders and shoulder blades form the base of a pyramid. Your head is the summit and your neck the center line leading to it. To complete the pyramid, all you have to do is draw a line from the top of your head to each side of the base line. The placement of your shoulders is determined by the degree of tension along these imaginary lines. With this system, you will easily see whether your neck and head are centered and whether your shoulders need adjustment.

1 Sit on the edge of a chair, back straight. Pull both shoulders up as if to touch your ears. Hold.
2 While holding, drop your chin onto your chest, so your head is down. Hold.

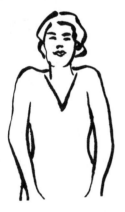 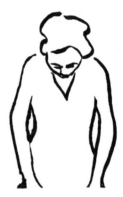

3 Gently bring your shoulders down and slowly bring your head
   back up. Relax.
Do three times.

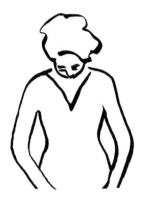 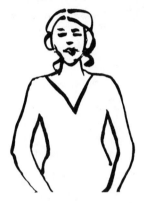

Practice Lab: Freeing Shoulders

1 Sit on the edge of a chair, keeping your back straight. Raise your right shoulder as high as you can, without moving your head/neck axis or your other shoulder. Hold. Relax.
2 Lower your right shoulder. Hold. Relax.
3 Raise your left shoulder. Hold. Relax.
4 Lower your left shoulder. Hold. Relax.

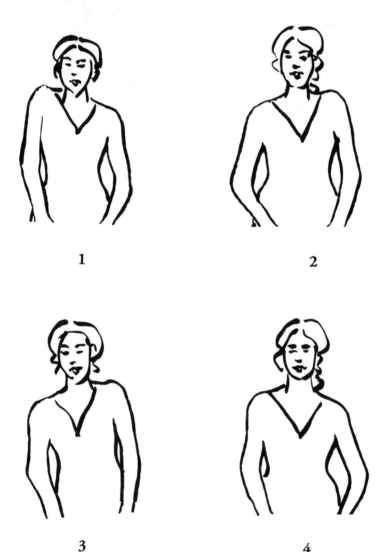

1   2

3   4

5 Push right shoulder forward. Hold. Relax.
6 Push left shoulder forward. Hold. Relax.
7 Push right shoulder back. Hold. Relax.
8 Push left shoulder back. Hold. Relax.
Do four times.

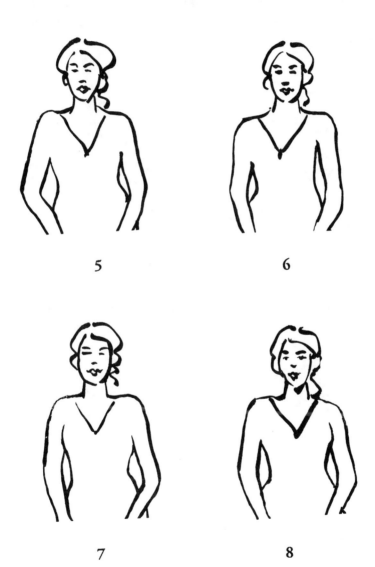

5

6

7

8

Practice Lab: Freeing Head/Neck

1 Slowly as you exhale, drop your chin down. Hold to the count of four. As you are ready to inhale, bring your head up.
2 Gently, as you exhale, drop your head backward. Hold four. As you are ready to inhale, bring your head straight up. Relax.
3 Lower your head to the right side, as if to touch your right shoulder the duration of one exhalation. Slowly bring your head straight up as you inhale.

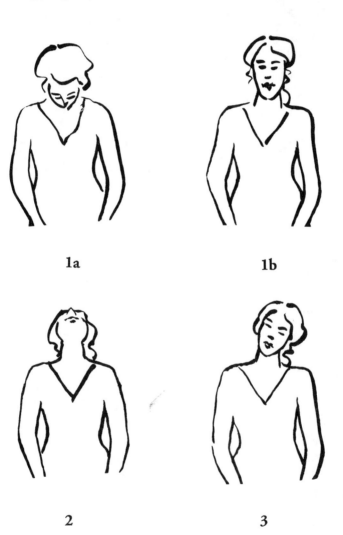

1a   1b

2   3

4 With care, lower your head to the left side as if to touch your left shoulder. Hold for the duration of one exhalation. Slowly bring your head straight up as you inhale. Relax.

5 Allowing your breathing to be open and free, turn your head to the right as far as you can go, looking over your right shoulder. Hold four counts.

6 Slowly bring your head back to center, then turn your head to the left as far as you can, looking over your left shoulder. Hold four. Slowly bring your head to the center.

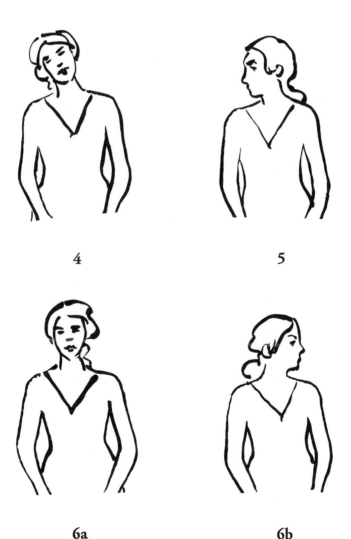

4

5

6a

6b

Practice Lab: Head Circles

1 Sit on the edge of a chair, keeping your back straight. Slowly turn your head to the right.

2 Looking as far as you can over your right shoulder, drop your chin toward your shoulder. Draw a half-circle on your chest going toward your left until your head is aligned over your left shoulder. Repeat to the right.

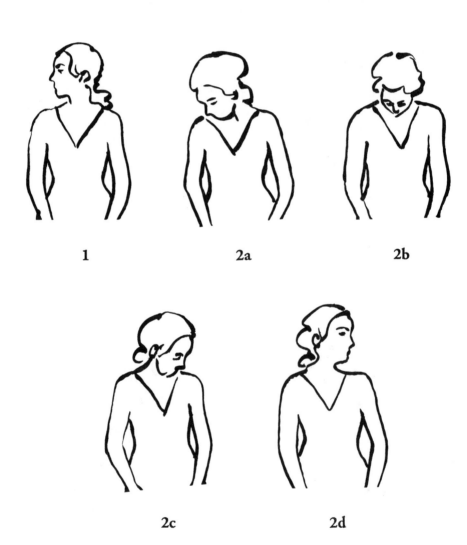

1   2a   2b

2c   2d

3 Turn your head to the left, raising your chin high enough to draw a half-circle clockwise, until your chin almost touches your right shoulder.

4 Retrace your steps, chin up, moving toward your left until your chin almost touches your left shoulder.

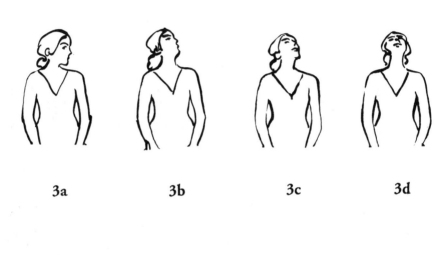

3a 3b 3c 3d

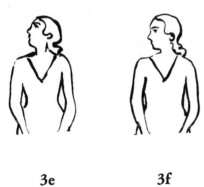

3e 3f

5 Turn your head to the left, raise your chin up, slowly drawing a half-circle toward your right. Drop your chin down to meet your right shoulder and continue going clockwise drawing a half-circle on your chest until your chin almost touches your left shoulder. Slowly retrace your steps the same way to complete a full-circle counter-clockwise.

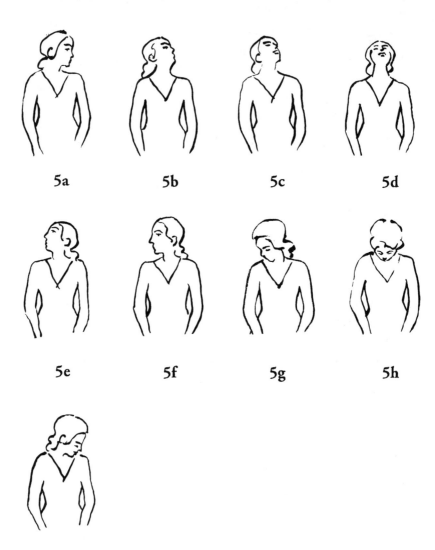

5a   5b   5c   5d

5e   5f   5g   5h

5i

Practice Lab: Back Roll

Sit on the edge of a chair, keeping your back erect. Drop your chin and head down onto your chest, then curl your shoulders forward. Gradually drop your torso down until your head is between your knees and your chest is rolled onto your lap. Take a deep breath in, then exhale fully. Inhale and slowly roll your spine up, making sure your shoulders come first, then your neck and finally your head. Relax.

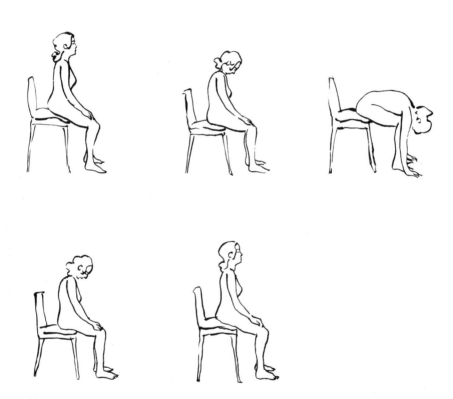

Summary

Limbering up your joints regularly prevents stiffness and accidents. Your legs and feet are like the foundation of a building. Keeping them fit guarantees the good condition of the whole. Your head, neck and shoulders relate to one another along the spinal axis. Keeping them adjusted is necessary in order to prevent tension. Your gait is determined by the dynamic relationship between pelvis, legs and spine.

Thought for the Day

Your living organism is your own precious instrument. Why not tune it well before every performance?

STEP SEVEN
Your Weekly Workout

When I moved to New York City in the late sixties, I was invited to teach privately in the salon of Elizabeth Arden. When I reported to work that first Monday morning, I was handed a list of my appointments for the day. The first one read, *Miss Gardner.* "She is waiting for you in your studio," the receptionist said.

I recognized her immediately, even though she was sprawled across the floor, warming up in the wake of her lesson. Ava Gardner! I had read about her love affairs, her life in Spain, her love of parties and the way she loved to dance flamenco all night. But it was the myth of her legendary beauty that was in my mind at that moment of instant recognition. I was stunned. It was important that I be discreet and respect her anonymity, which was her wish, but I had to contain myself.

We worked together for an hour. She moved beautifully and unhurriedly. I could see that she loved to stretch the way cats do, taking her time, sensuously feeling the stretch all the way through. What made her movements remarkable was that she gave the impression that nothing was more important than what she was doing at that very moment. As a result, her simplest gesture had a smoothness that made it beautiful. Hers was an attitude of simplicity and intention of purpose, not one of having to achieve a goal at any cost. She was like the swimmer who enjoys riding with the waves, for she was always economizing her energy, letting go before and after exertion.

It was a lesson for me that beauty is in the vitality released through movement—the question was how to bring it to the surface. Could stretching be the answer?

I have long been aware that we can maintain a high level of tone (readiness for action in muscle tissue). Stretching is nature's way of allowing this to happen, for when we stretch, we enter the animal kingdom by becoming a cat, a dog or a horse. Birds, too, have a funny way of stretching their necks as they shake them in all directions. In stretching, we rediscover our natural heritage. We become fully creatures of the earth.

What can a good stretch do for you? It mobilizes energy and keeps the muscles resilient. When you release the stretch, blood flow accelerates in the muscular tissues and waste products are removed.

Before you can stretch properly, you have to understand how your muscles function. As discussed previously, your bones form your structural framework. Imagine how your body would feel without bones. If you did not have bones, gravity would make pulp of you!

A muscle is a unit of fibrous tissue that has the capacity to contract and relax. Muscles organize themselves around your bones with the help of ligaments and tendons and extend the freedom of movement already given by the joints.

Your muscles work in pairs—agonist and antagonist. When one stretches, the other flexes; it is a marriage of cooperation for life. For your system to be well-balanced, a pair of muscles has to pull equally in its appropriate direction. Remember the diagram in Step Six that showed how the units that come in pairs around your frame have to be equally balanced. Stretching helps to maintain the correct balance.

Muscle tone refers to the firmness of the muscles while in repose. A muscle does not lose its tone when at rest, as long as rest does not mean chronic passivity. There is no such thing as complete repose, only a lower rate of metabolic interchange. Connective tissue is in a constant state of re-organization.

Your strongest muscles are your back muscles. The most important of these are three long muscles that originate at the base of the spine and attach themselves to the base of the skull. They enable you to stand. They are paired with the long abdominal muscles which attach the fifth rib to the pubic bone. When the back muscles extend, the abdominal muscles flex.

The psoas muscle is the most important of the abdominal muscles because of its direct influence on the diaphragm, spine, pelvis and femur. Attached to the last dorsal and first lumbar vertebrae, it comes down obliquely through the pelvic structure and crosses over the pubic bone, ending up joined to the upper femur. If you realize how the diaphragm influences breathing, then you will easily see how crucial the elasticity of the abdominal wall is to your health.

Muscles in your legs and pelvis allow forward and backward movement, rotation and sideways movement. Muscles in your arms allow forward and backward motion, flexing and extending, rotation and up-and-down movement. These movements play an important part in your Workout Program.

You need to do the Tune-up in Step Six before you begin your

Workout. When the Workout Program has been completely established in your life, then it will be required only once a week as your daily Maintenance Program (Step Eight) will take precedence.

Workout Program

Your Workout Program is to be learned progressively over a period of three weeks. I have divided it into one-week segments so that by the third week you will do the complete Workout.

The first week, which I will refer to from now on as Section A, will include a daily regimen of stretches for the health and tone of your back and abdomen.

The second week you will practice, in addition to the Practice Labs in Section A, the stretches in Section B, which flex and tone your limbs.

The third week you will practice Sections A and B plus Section C—stretches to center and balance you spatially.

Together these three stretches form not only a thorough shape-up program, but also a preparation for the sensuous awakening dance sequence which you will start on the fifth week and which will become your essential daily tool for staying in shape. After the fourth week, Sections A, B and C, plus the Tune-up Program in Step Six, will be used as a support program once a week.

Section A—Week I

This section includes six movements done in a combination to be repeated four times. These are excellent therapy for your back and abdomen. Each is on a 4/4 rhythm, which means that you either hold the movement for four counts or relax for four counts. Once you have done these six movements, you repeat the whole segment three more times. In all, you will have done the same combination four times. Section A, once learned, should only take ten minutes. Center yourself with Tool 1 and pay attention to your breathing. Unless indicated otherwise, adjust your breathing to what is comfortable for you.

Practice Lab: Section A, Movement 1

1 Lie on your back, knees bent, both feet on the floor, arms along
  your sides.
2 With both hands, bring your right knee up over your chest,
  keeping your back and shoulders flat against the floor. Hold
  for four counts. Bring your foot down.
3 Alternate legs.
Do each leg four times.

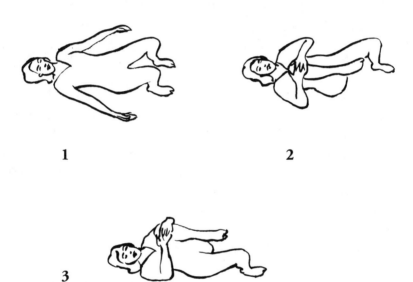

1   2

3

Practice Lab: Section A, Movement 2

Your posture and the flatness of your stomach depend on the psoas muscles which work in sync with the rectus abdomini.

1 Stay on your back, both knees bent, feet on the floor. Press the small of your back against the floor, pulling your abdominal muscles and buttocks in tight. Hold to the count of four.
2 Relax to the count of four.
Do four times.

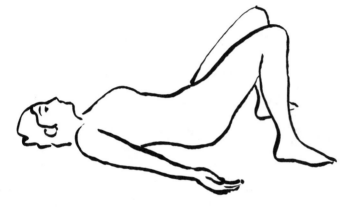

Practice Lab: Section A, Movement 3

This is another one to condition your back.

1 Stay on your back. With both hands, bring both knees up and bend them over your chest. Bring your knees as close to your chest as you can. Hold four counts.

2 Relax four counts.

Do four times.

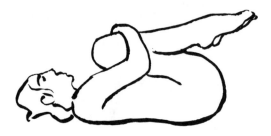

1

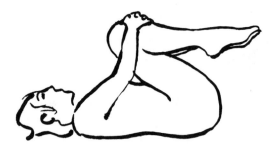

2

Practice Lab: Section A, Movement 4

This is an excellent tightener for your midriff and stomach area.

1 Stay on your back, with knees bent over the chest, both hands clasped firmly behind your head.
2 As you exhale, bring your left elbow to touch your right knee. Bring your head back down, inhale.
3 As you exhale, bring your right elbow to touch your left knee, then your head to the floor and inhale.

Do four times, both sides.

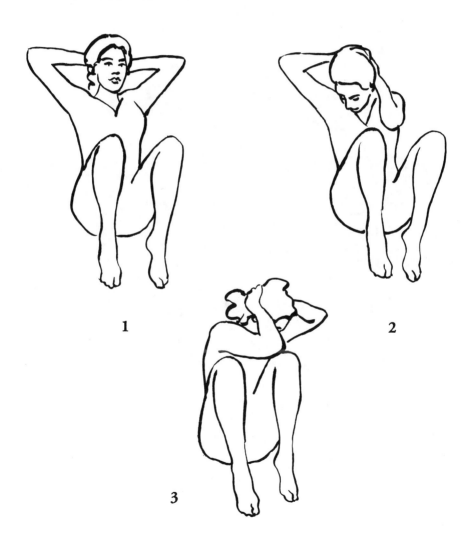

1

2

3

Practice Lab: Section A, Movement 5

This movement relates to the psoas unit. It conditions and tones your back and abdomen.

1 Stay on your back. Bend your knees with feet wide apart on the floor. Press the small of your back against the floor, and as you tilt your pelvis up, raise your hips off the floor and arch your back as high as you can so only your shoulders touch the floor. Stay up for four counts.
2 Roll down, upper spine first, then middle spine, and last the small of the back touches the floor.

Do four times.

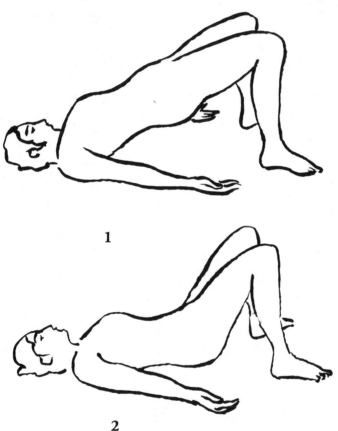

1

2

Practice Lab: Section A, Movement 6

This helps to tone your abdomen.

1 Stay on your back, knees bent, feet on the floor, hands clasped behind your head. As you exhale, bring your head and upper torso up. Hold for four counts.

2 Bring your head back to the floor, inhale. Rest for four counts. Do four times.

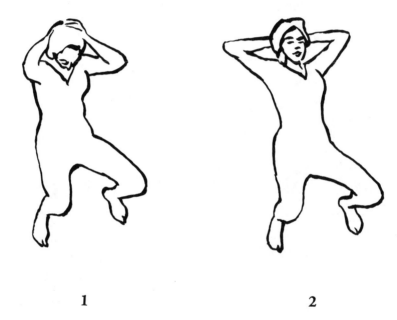

1   2

Repeat entire Section A three more times.

Section B—Week II

Your daily Workout will now include Section A plus Section B—stretches for the health and tone of your limbs. Section B includes 7 movements. Unless indicated otherwise, adjust your breathing to what feels comfortable. Once learned, Section B should take no more than 10 minutes.

Practice Lab: Section B, Movement 1

Movement 1 will shape your thighs and legs, as well as maintain their flexibility. Note that the number of times required for each exercise varies.

1 Lie on your back, arms outstretched, knees bent, feet together on the floor.
2 Bend your right knee and bring it over your chest and flex your right foot.

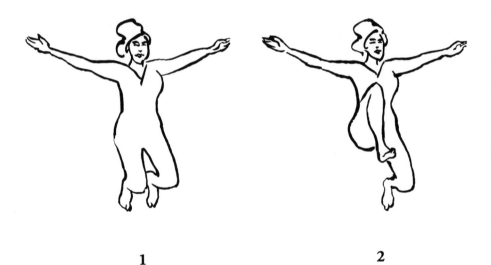

1   2

3 Extend your right leg upward, foot pointed toward ceiling.
4 In an open movement, bring your right leg as far to the side as
   you can.
5 Keeping your right leg opened out, bend your right knee so
   your right foot moves inward toward your crotch and flex your
   foot.

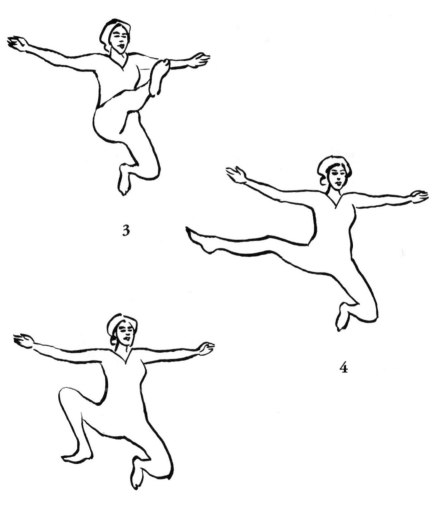

3

4

5

6 Bring your right knee up over your chest, keeping your right foot flexed. Repeat Movements 3—6.

Do each leg four times.

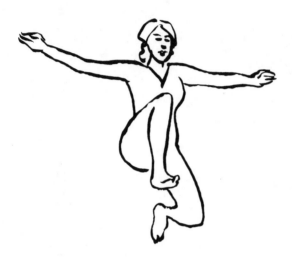

Practice Lab: Section B, Movement 2

This will reduce and tone your hips. Stay on your back, knees bent over chest, feet off the floor, arms outstretched.

1 Keeping the knees together, drop them to the floor on your right.
2 From the floor, extend both legs straight out, toes pointed.
3 Bend both knees and bring them up and over your chest.

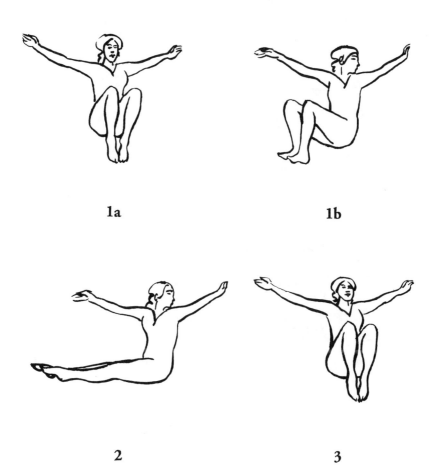

1a   1b

2   3

4 Keeping the knees together, drop them to the floor on your left.

5 From the floor, extend both legs straight out, toes pointed.

6 Bend both knees and bring them up and over your chest.

Do routine 5 times.

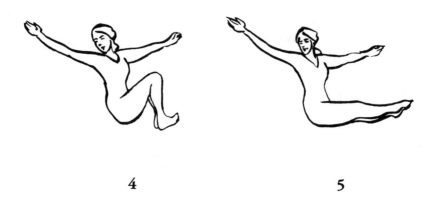

4   5

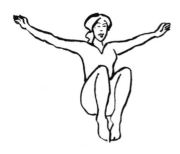

6

Practice Lab: Section B, Movement 3

Movement 3 will tone the inner and outer part of your arms and legs.

Fold a towel in four and make a roll out of it. Place it under the base of your spine for support and extend both arms and legs straight up toward the ceiling.

1 Turn your arms and legs inward so your fingertips and toes touch.
2 Spread your arms and legs open, keeping your fingers and toes turned in.

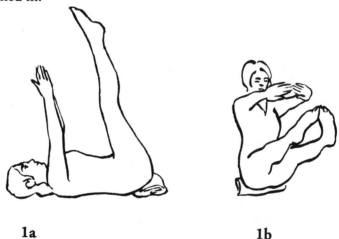

1a **1b**

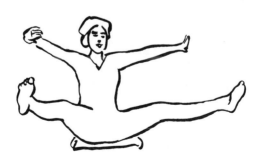

2

3 Slowly turn your arms and legs out while staying in the open position.
4 Without changing the turn-out, bring them together so your wrists and heels come together.

Do routine 10 times.

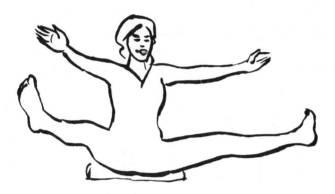

3

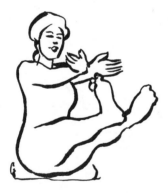

4

Practice Lab: Section B, Movement 4

This movement will give tone to arms and legs as well as reinforce the tone of the abdominal muscles.

1 Stay on your back, both knees bent over your chest, palms together as though you were diving, elbows bent.
2 Straighten both arms and legs up toward the ceiling.

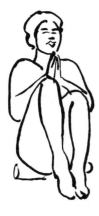

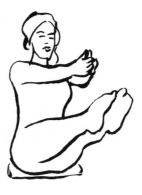

1   **2**

3 Spread both legs and arms straight open toward the sides.
4 Bend your knees and elbows together as you bring your knees
and joined hands over your chest. Do four times.

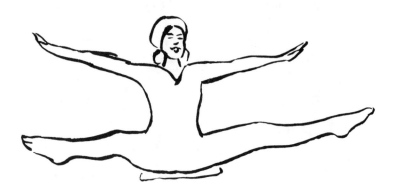

3

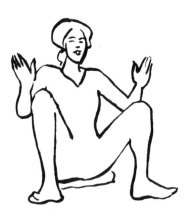

4a

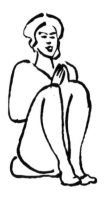

4b

Practice Lab: Section B, Movement 5

This movement is the reverse of Movement 4.

1 Stay on your back, knees bent together over your chest, hands joined together.
2 Extend both arms and legs straight out in a V position.

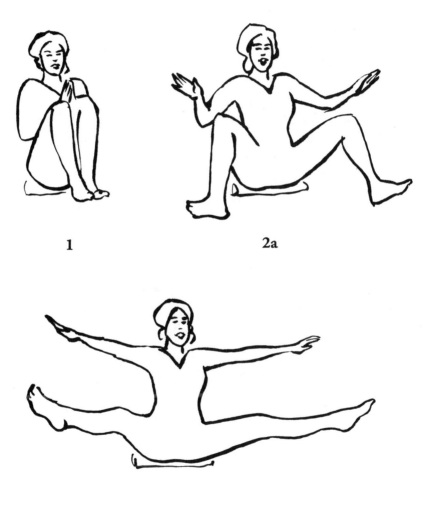

1   2a

2b

3 Bring both arms and legs straight together over your chest so
  they point toward the ceiling.
4 Bend both knees and arms toward your chest as your hands join
  together. Do four times.

Repeat Movements 4 and 5.

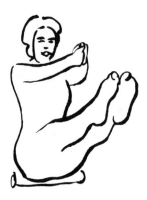

3

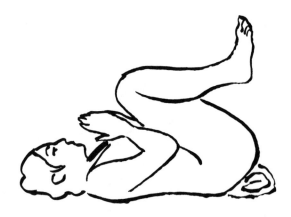

4

Practice Lab: Section B, Movement 6

Movements 6 and 7 are my favorite stretches. They act as a tonic for the whole body. Through contraction and extension, these stretches involve full action of flexors and extensors in an agonist/antagonist interplay.

1 Turn on your right side, leaning on your right forearm. Your right knee is on the floor, flexed in front of you. Your left leg is extended alongside on the floor.
2 Pointing your left knee toward the ceiling, bring it toward your forehead, using the help of your left arm. Exhale.

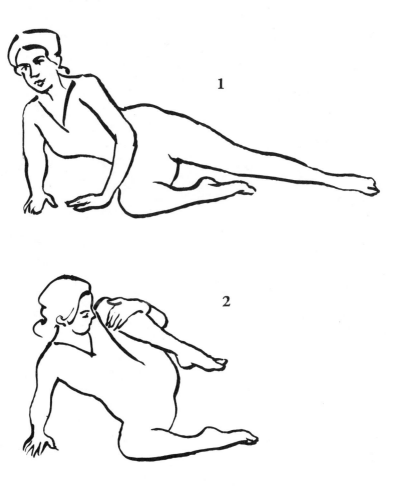

3 Inhaling, stretch your left arm and leg fully, along the line of your body.

4 Stretch your left arm up and around in a wheel as your knee begins to contract. You are again at number 2.
Perform eight times.

Repeat on left side eight times.

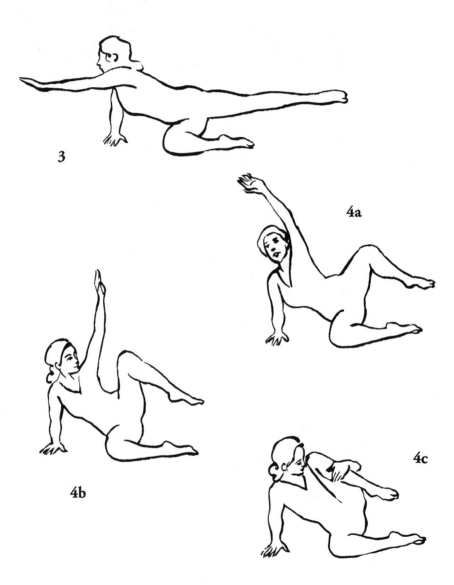

3

4a

4b

4c

Practice Lab: Section B, Movement 7

1 Get on your hands and knees.
2 Bring your right knee and your head toward each other.
3 Raise your head and stretch out your right leg behind you as
   high as you can.
4 Bend your knee, flexing your foot.
5 Extend your right leg once more with your toes pointed.
6 Return your right knee to the floor.

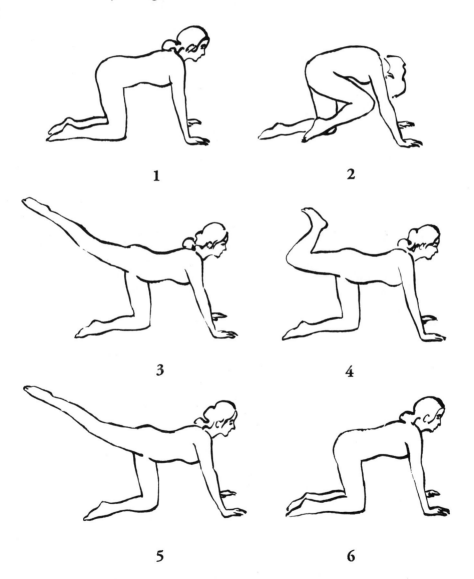

7 Bring your left knee and your head toward each other.
8 Raise your head and stretch out your left leg behind you as high as you can.
9 Bend your knee, flexing your foot.
10 Extend your left leg once more with your toes pointed.
11 Return your left knee to the floor.
Do each leg four times.
Do routine twice.

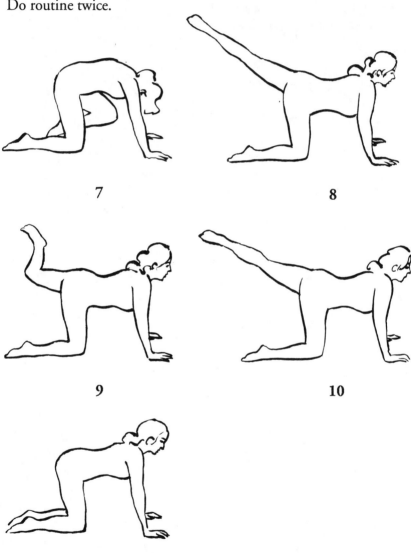

7

8

9

10

11

Section C—Week III

Your daily Workout will now include Section A, Section B and Section C (stretches for centering and balance control). When you have learned them, they will take no more than 25 minutes of your time. Section C includes three movements. Adjust your breathing according to how it feels.

Practice Lab: Section C, Movement 1

With this movement you practice centering.

1 Stand up, feet together, arms along your sides.
2 Flex your knees as you exhale, keeping your back straight.
3 As you inhale, straighten your legs. Flex your elbows as you lift your arms to the sides like a swan slowly stretching out its wings.

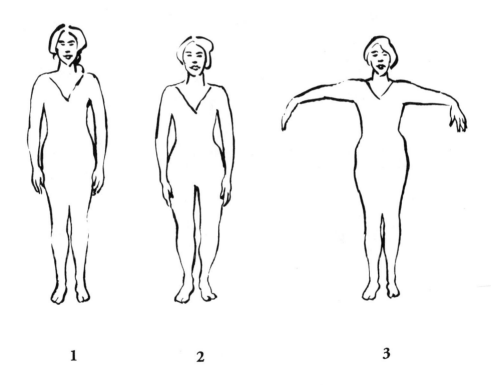

1   2   3

4 Raise yourself on tiptoe as your arms continue going up. Keep
your balance, tightening your abdominal muscles, until your
hands join above your head. The tighter you pull in your
abdomen, the more centered and balanced you are.

5 As you exhale, turn your hands out and slowly lower your arms
as you bring your heels down. Relax. Do four times.

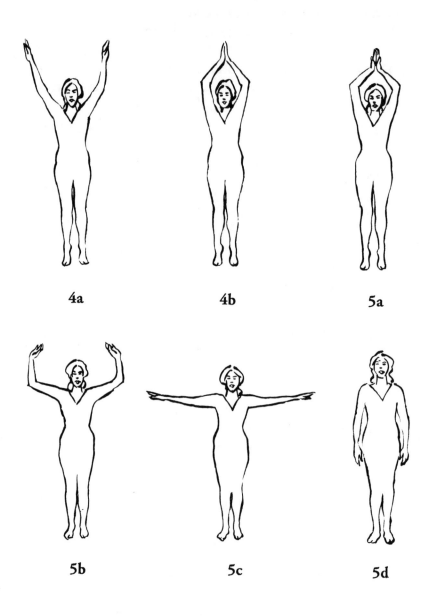

4a   4b   5a

5b   5c   5d

Practice Lab: Section C, Movement 2

Movement 2 is for balance control as well as for centering.

1 Stand, feet together, arms along your sides.
2 Keeping your back straight, flex your knees as you inhale. Raise
   your arms straight in front of you on a horizontal plane and
   join your palms.
3 On the outbreath, turn your hands out.

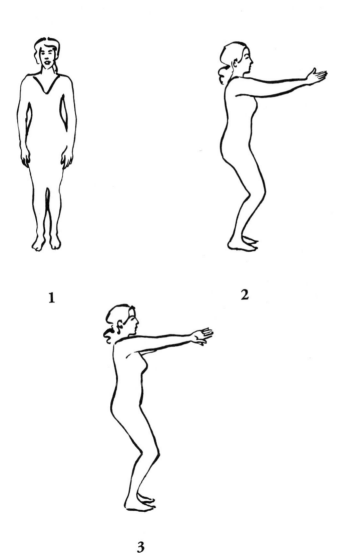

1

2

3

4 Inhaling, raise yourself on tiptoe and push your arms out to the sides.

5 Exhale, lowering heels and relaxing arms along your sides.

Do four times.

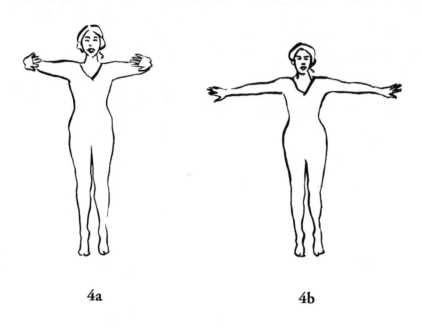

4a   4b

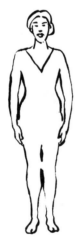

5

Practice Lab: Section C, Movement 3

This movement refines balance control and helps develop command over self.

1 Stand up, feet together, arms along your sides. Shift your weight to your left side.
2 Pick up your right knee with both hands and bring it up as high as possible.

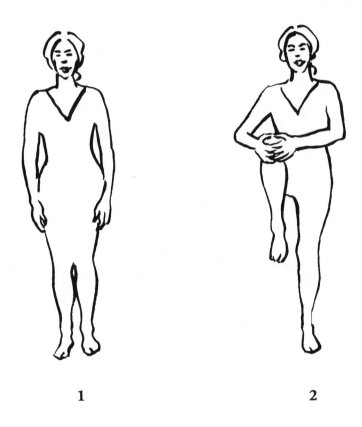

1   2

3 Slowly lower your arms to your sides and your right leg back to the floor so your body weight is equally supported by both legs.
4 Shift your weight to your left side.

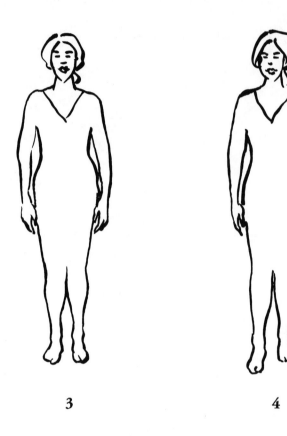

3   4

5 Catch your right foot behind you with your right hand (the knee is bent). Find your balance as you stand.

6 Still standing on your left leg, slowly bend forward, extending your left arm in front of you, left wrist bent. Holding your right foot behind you, pull it up as high as you can.

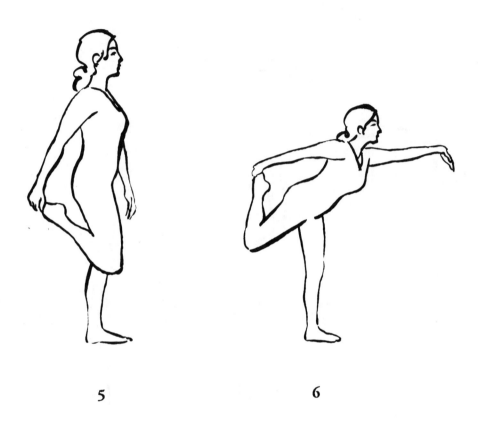

5   6

7 Slowly move your left hand in line with the extended left arm and extend both right arm and leg straight behind you. Hold your balance as long as you can.

8 Relax, bringing your foot back to the floor and arms back to your sides.

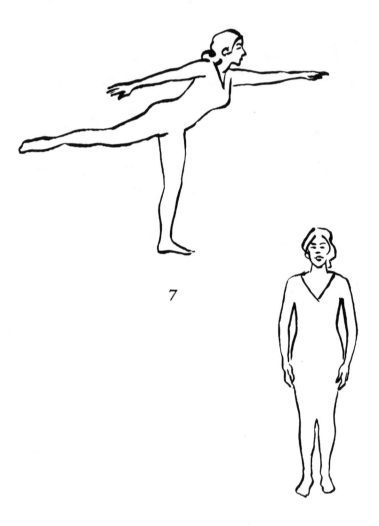

7

8

9 Stand up, feet together, arms along your sides. Shift your weight to your right side.

10 Pick up your left knee with both hands and bring it up as high as possible.

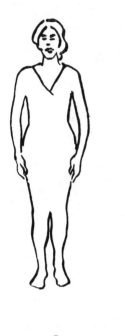

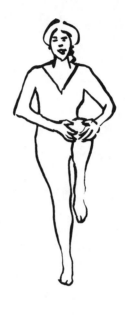

9   **10**

11 Slowly lower your arms to your sides and your left leg back to the floor so your body weight is equally supported by both legs.

12 Shift your weight to your right side.

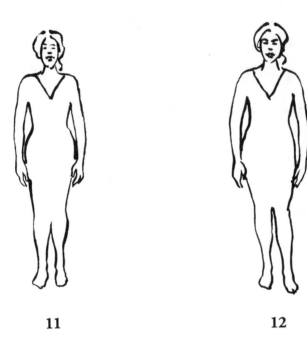

11   12

13 Catch your left foot behind you with your left hand (the knee is bent). Find your balance as you stand.

14 Still standing on your right leg, slowly bend forward, extending your right arm in front of you, right wrist bent. Holding your left foot behind you, pull it up as high as you can.

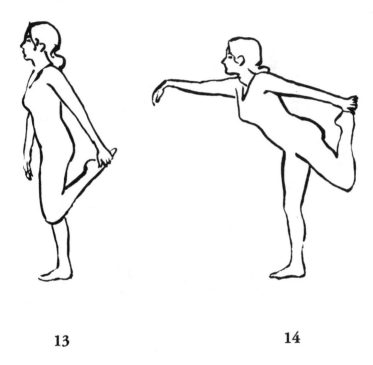

13   14

15 Slowly move your right hand in line with the extended right arm and extend both left arm and leg straight behind you. Hold your balance as long as you can.

16 Relax, bringing your foot back to the floor and arms back to your sides.

Do routine twice.

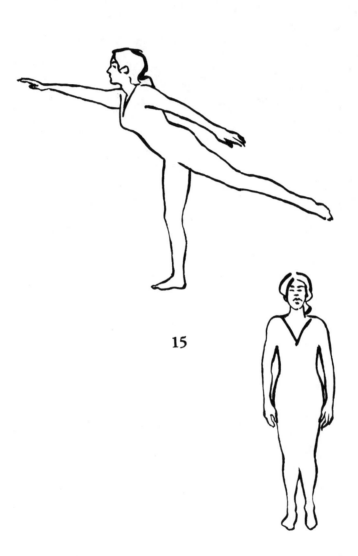

15

16

Summary

Stretching prepares you for activity, tuning each muscle group equally. Relaxing before and after a stretch will maximize the effect.

Your Workout Program is progressive. It is a three-week program of specific movements that concentrate on your back and abdomen first, then your limbs and ends with the emphasis on centering and balance.

Thought for the Day

Stretching is the gate to freedom and beauty.

STEP EIGHT
The Dance

Like the soil which needs nurturing in order to grow a fine crop, your body needs care. While we are young and healthy, we tend to take our looks and muscle tone for granted. But by middle-age we start to panic and wonder how we can regain what we have lost. We cannot stop the clock, but we can have it serviced! One way is to exercise. The myth about exercise is that sheer repetition will strengthen a muscle. The reality is that most often it upsets the reciprocal activity of the agonist-antagonist operation. The real benefits come from paying attention to the way it is done, rather than the exercise itself.

I call this Step "The Dance" because the sequence of movements is organized not only to provide dynamic muscular balance but also to entertain the mind. The Dance integrates everything you have learned so far.

You might wonder: why a dance? Dance is the medium of interrelated movements. In the Classic tradition of ballet, the art of dance is in the quality of flow that emanates between one movement and another. John Martin was a dance critic for the *New York Times* and author of *The Modern Dance*, a remarkable book in which he describes how movement becomes dance. He says, "Dance is not the series of connected postures, but rather the stuff that connects the postures together." Thus, the inherent beauty of a movement is underlined by a pause or breathing space before or after stretching.

Wouldn't you rather do a dance every morning to keep in shape? I know I would. It feels right. It charges my batteries as I feel the skin tighten around my muscles. Who wouldn't like it?

Your dance lasts seven minutes. Who has seven minutes to spare? Everybody, including you.

Bridges

Make sure before you begin that you have at least the space of a body length in front of and behind you and the width of your outstretched arms. The Bridges and The Dance require more space than the other Practice Labs.

I call a Bridge a point in the sequence that provides new spatial orientation. There are three Bridges in the sequence. Each day for one week, practice each one separately after you have finished your Tune-up Program and before you begin the dance sequence.

Bridge 1: Head Dive, Squat 'n Roll-up

1 Exhale as you flex your knees while keeping your heels firmly to the ground. Drop your chin onto your chest as your head moves down, followed by your shoulders. Flex your knees even more to release tension in your back. Now you are bent from the waist down.
2 Place your hands flat on the floor in front of you. Bend your knees and move forward, allowing your heels to come up naturally.

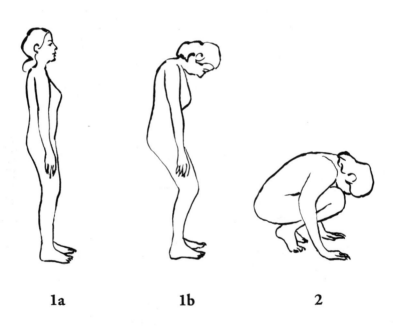

1a   1b   2

3 Inhaling, sit on your heels as you straighten your spine and
  bring up your head. Allow your hands to slide backward to your
  sides.
4 Exhale, drop your head once more into your knees and place
  your hands flat on the floor in front of you.
5 Keeping your head down, drop your heels and slowly straighten
  your legs. Gradually straighten your spine.
Do three times.

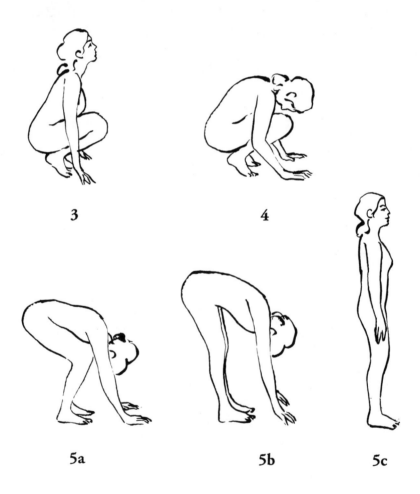

3   4

5a   5b   5c

Bridge 2: Sit-Ups

This Bridge is a marvelous toner for your back and abdominal muscles. Remember that your back muscles work in tandem with your abdominal muscles.

1 Sit down on the floor, keeping your knees bent and your feet flat on the floor. Extend your arms in front of you and drop your chin onto your chest.

2 Using your extended arms as a balancing device, slowly roll down your spine until you are lying on the floor. Your arms are relaxed along your sides.

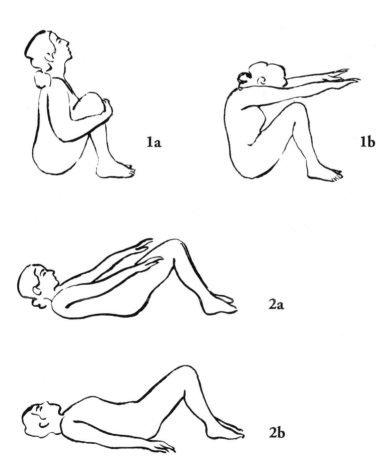

1a

1b

2a

2b

3 Press the base of your back firmly into the floor and with both arms stretched forward, come up again in a sitting position.

Do six times; increase to 10 and eventually to 15. You might need help at first. If you do, place your feet under a sofa or have a friend hold your feet firmly down.

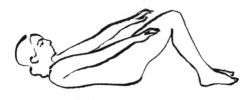

3a

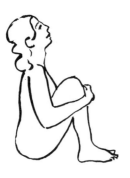

3b

Bridge 3: Sit, Squat 'n Kneel

If you are doing your sit-ups easily, your back has enough strength to work on the third Bridge. Move to Bridge 3 only when you are confident with Bridge 2. Bridge 3 helps you practice transferring weight from a sitting position to a position on all fours in the dance sequence.

1 Sit down on the floor, knees bent and feet down. Place your hands on the floor behind your hips, turning your hands around so that your thumbs point forward and your fingers backward.
2 With the help of your hands, push yourself forward lifting your heels. Your knees move forward while your head and shoulders fall back. Take a deep breath in.
3 Reverse back to the first position. Exhale.
Do four times.

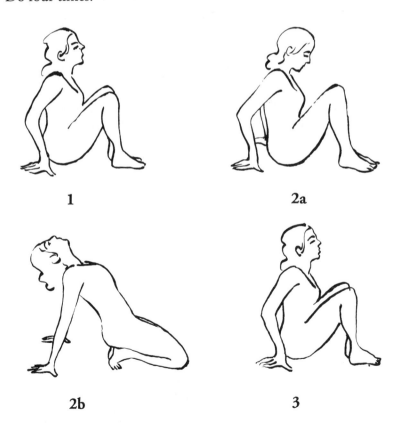

1   2a

2b   3

The Dance

Your dance is organized around 88 moves. The end of one move is the beginning of the next. When you do the sequence, keep in mind that you must progress through it at an even pace. The same speed is to be maintained all the way through.

Although breathing directions are given only when necessary, be attentive to your breath at all times, as it will guide you in achieving fluid movements. Place your attention on your navel. (You will find out why in Step Nine). Your emotions and thoughts—your self awareness—will affect the quality of your movements. When you get to the end, you are right back where you started—at the beginning.

Every day of the fifth week after you have done the Tune-up and worked on the three Bridges, go over about ten of the Dance Moves. By the end of the week, you will have practiced all of them. In the sixth week you are ready to do the Dance every day plus a complete Workout once a week. If you are not ready, continue with the preliminary practice in this Step until you are ready.

1 Feet together, relax both shoulders, letting your arms hang freely.

2 Exhale slowly as you flex your knees over your feet.

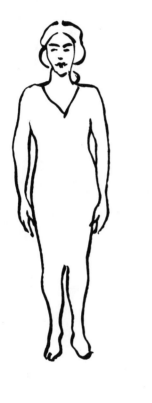

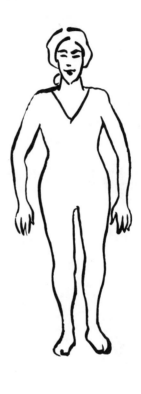

1

2

3 Slowly raise arms straight in front of you, wrists relaxed.
4 Bring hands into alignment with arms.
5 Return to position 1.
6 Inhaling, flex your elbows as you lift your arms to the sides like
   a swan slowly stretching out its wings.

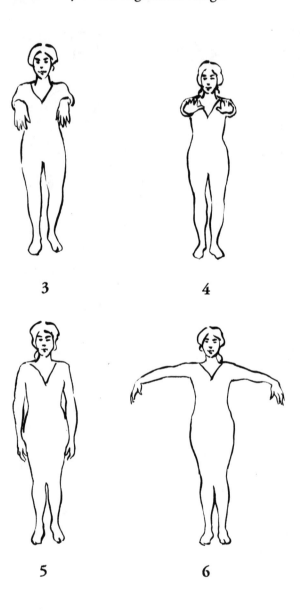

3

4

5

6

7 Raise yourself on tiptoe as your arms continue going up. Join
your palms above your head.
8 Maintain your balance by pulling up every fiber in your being.
Turn your palms out.
9 Slowly lower your arms as you flex your knees.
10 Drop your head onto your chest.

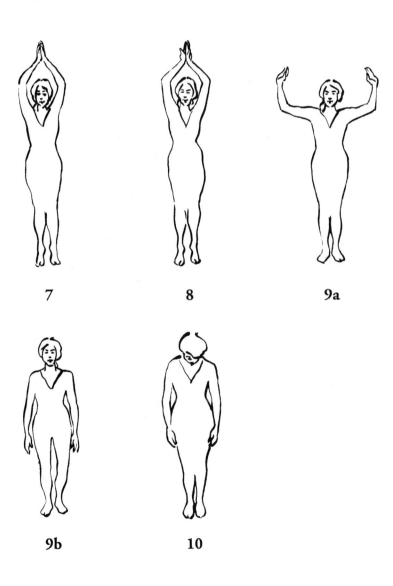

7   8   9a

9b   10

11 Curl your shoulders in and slowly roll your spine down as you bend your knees.

12 Place your hands on the floor and squat with your heels raised. Raise your head.

13 Bring your hands behind you on either side of your hips, thumbs facing forward.

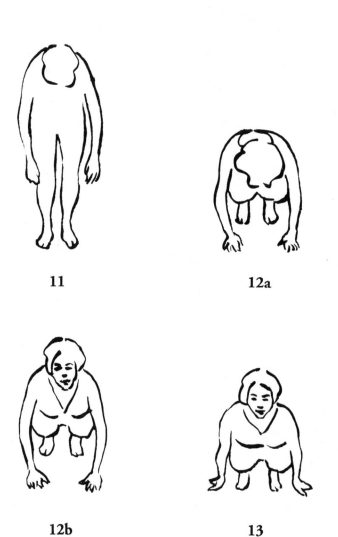

11   12a

12b   13

14 Extend your right leg straight out from under you.

15 Do the same with the left. Both legs are now extended in front of you as you support yourself with your hands.

16 Sit down and extend your arms straight out in front of you.

17 Drop your chin onto your chest and roll your spine slowly onto the floor until you are lying fully stretched.

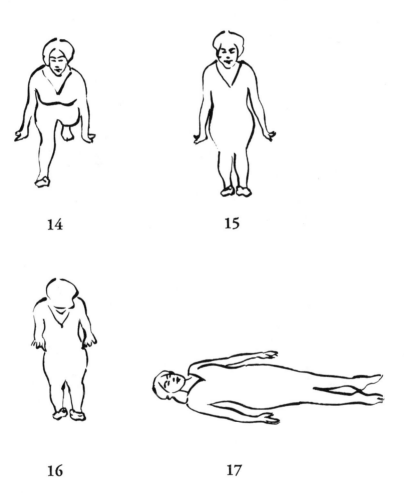

14   15

16   17

18 Bring your right knee to your chest with both hands.

19 Drop your arms open in a sensing and flowing way.

20 Cross your right knee toward your left side, pulling your right hip off the floor as you turn your head in the opposite direction.

21 Bring your right knee and your head back to center.

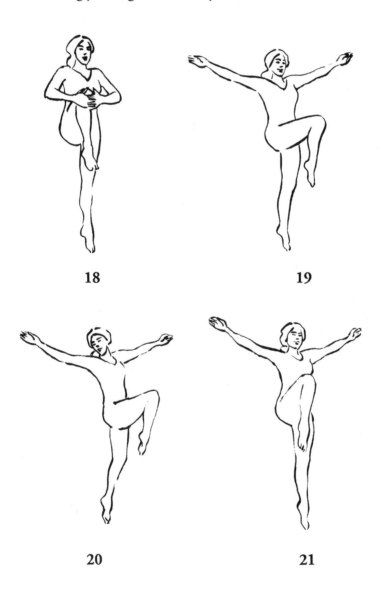

18

19

20

21

22 Drop your right knee to your right side and flex your foot.

23 Stretch your leg straight out as though you were giving a kick, pointing your toes.

24 Slide your leg along the floor, bringing your arms down your sides in a sensuous way. Take a moment to feel the openness in your chest where you feel your breath come and go.

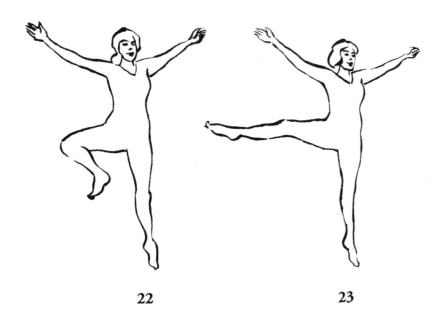

22   23

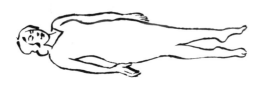

24

25 Bring your left knee to your chest with both hands.

26 Drop your arms open in a sensing and flowing way.

27 Cross your left knee toward your right side, pulling your left hip off the floor as you turn your head in the opposite direction.

28 Bring your left knee and your head back to center.

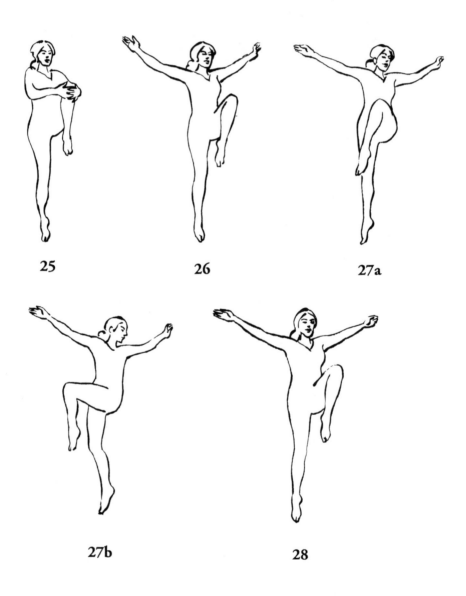

25   26   27a

27b   28

29 Drop your left knee to your left side and flex your foot.

30 Stretch your leg straight out as though you were giving a kick, pointing your toes.

31 Slide your leg along the floor, bringing your arms down your sides in a sensuous way. Take a moment to feel the openness in your chest where you feel your breath come and go.

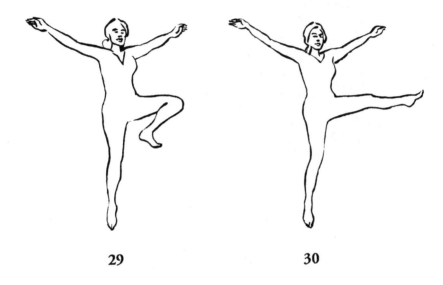

29   30

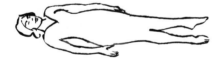

31

32 Exhale as you bring your knees to your chest, circling your arms around them. Your shoulders are flat on the floor.

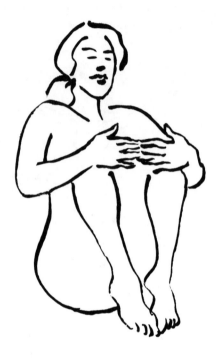

32

33 As you open your arms onto the floor, turn your head to the right and drop both knees to your left, flexing your feet.
34 Extend your legs straight out, pointing your toes.
35 Bend the knees and bring them back over your chest and your head to center.

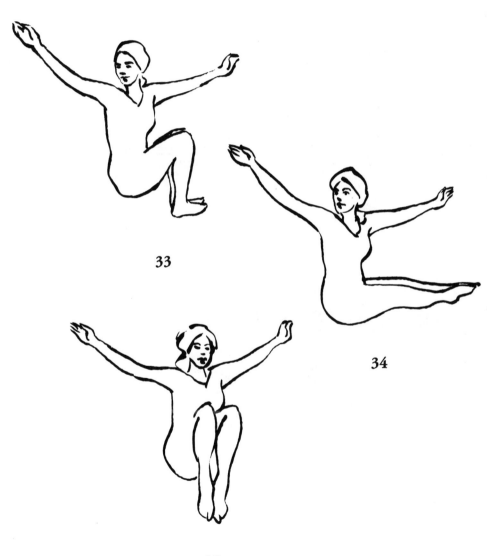

33

34

35

36 Turning your head to the left, drop both knees to your right, flexing your feet.

37 Extend your legs straight out, pointing your toes.

38 Bend the knees and bring them back over your chest and your head to center.

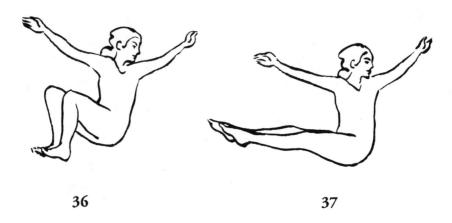

36   37

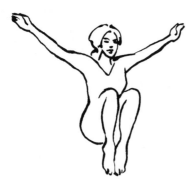

38

39 Bring your head to your knees, circling your arms around, and exhale deeply.

40 Bring your head back to the floor.

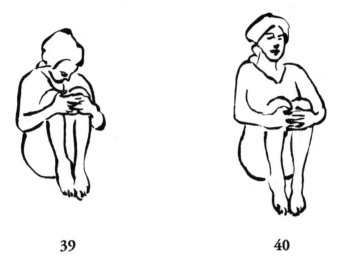

39   40

41 Drop your feet onto the floor, keeping your knees bent. Keeping elbows relaxed, bring the circle of your arms over and behind your head.

42 Bend your right knee over your chest and flex your foot.

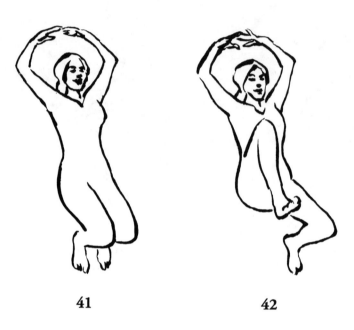

41   42

43 Extend your leg straight toward the ceiling, pointing your toes.

44 As you pull your stomach in, lower your right leg and sensuously slide your arms down along the floor.

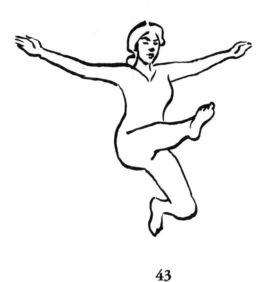

43

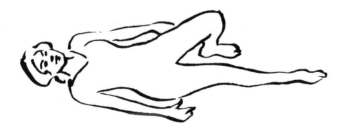

44

45 Bending the knee, place your right foot next to the left.
46 Bend your left knee over your chest, flexing your foot and bring the circle of your arms over and behind your head.

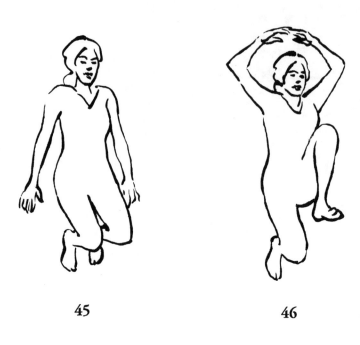

45   **46**

47 Extend your left leg straight up toward the ceiling, pointing your toes.

48 As you tighten your abdomen, lower your left leg and sensuously slide your arms down along the floor.

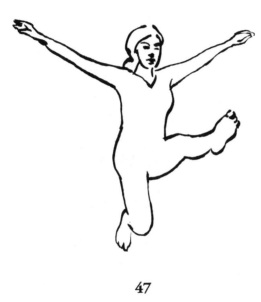

47

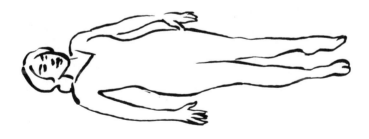

48

49 Bend the knee, and place your left foot next to the right.

50 Bring your head and knees together as you circle your arms around your knees. Exhale.

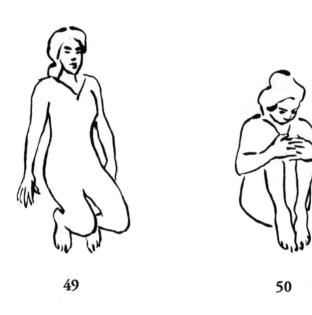

49   50

51 Bring your head back to the floor.

52 Extend both legs up toward the ceiling, pointing your toes.

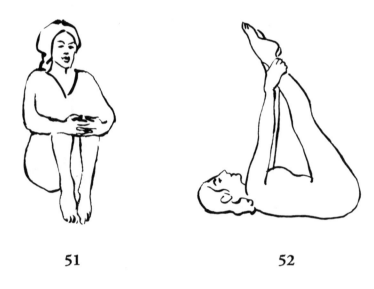

51   **52**

53 Take hold of your legs and bring your head to your knees. Exhale.

54 Bring your head back to the floor.

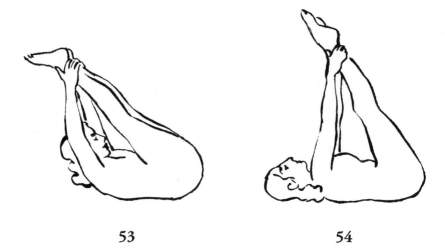

53   54

55 Keeping legs extended, place your hands between your knees and push your legs open.

56 Bend your knees and place your feet wide apart on the floor, arms relaxed along your body.

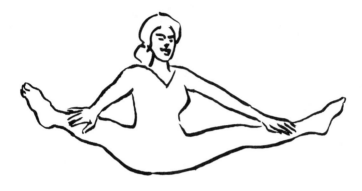

55

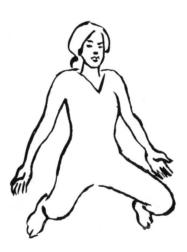

56

57 Press the small of your back against the floor and with your hands supporting your buttocks, start lifting both hips off the floor.

58 Push up, arching your back as much as you can without losing your balance.

59 Slowly roll your spine down to the floor until the lower spine comes to rest on the floor.

60 Bring your feet together.

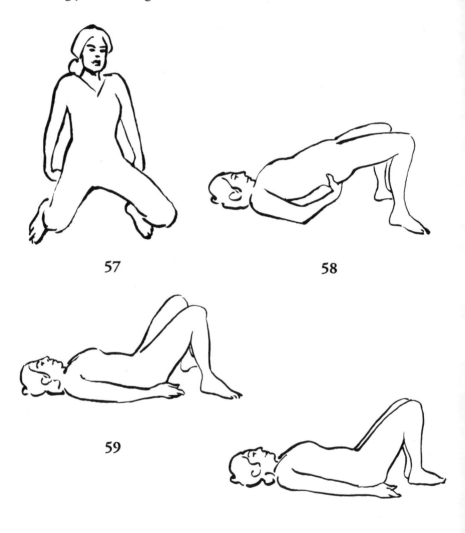

57

58

59

60

61 Press the small of your back against the floor as you thrust your arms forward and come to a sitting position, arms circling your knees. Straighten your back, head and neck.

62 Relax your neck, spine and arms. Sensuously open your knees toward the floor and hold your feet with your hands. Exhaling, bring your head toward your toes, flexing your elbows outward.

63 Inhaling, roll your spine up, neck and head last. With the help of your hands, bring your knees together.

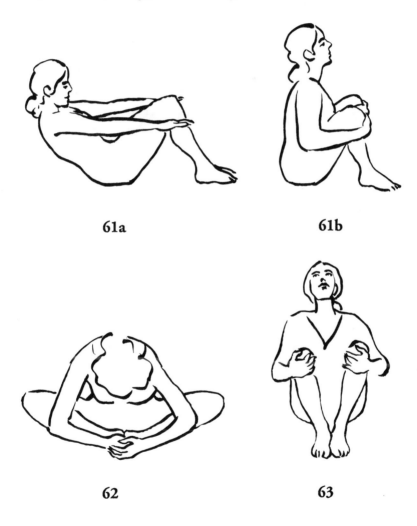

61a   61b

62   63

64 Relax your back and place your hands with thumbs facing forward on the floor behind your hips on either side.

65 Using your arms to give your body momentum, thrust your knees forward and allow your head to fall back as you arch your back. Take a deep breath in.

66 Slide your hands forward along your sides and squat, balancing your weight over your feet.

67 Place your hands in front of you and drop your knees. You are now on all fours.

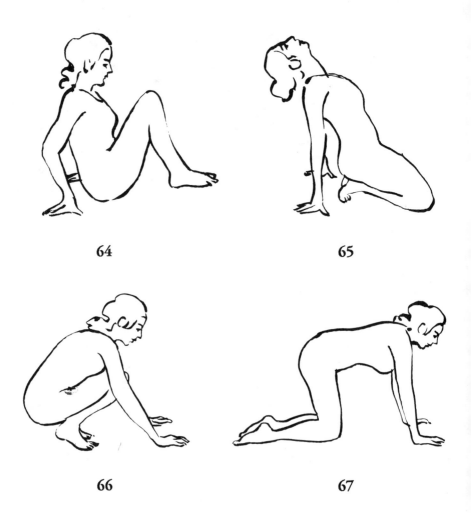

64

65

66

67

68 Exhaling, bring your right knee toward your forehead.
69 Gently raise your head and kick your right leg backward.

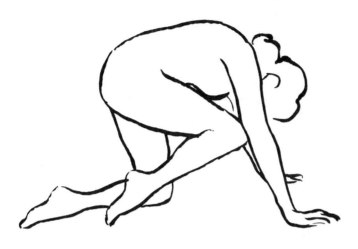

68

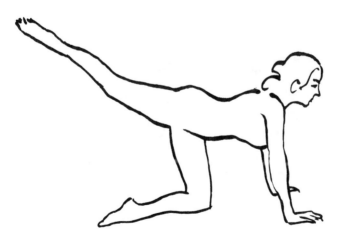

69

70 Keeping your right leg up, slowly flex your knee and foot.
71 Extend, pointing your toes.
72 Bring your right knee back to the floor.

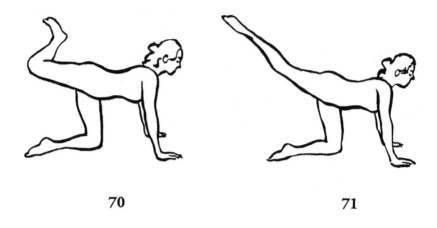

70

71

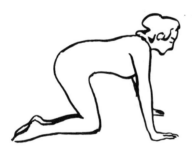

72

73 Exhaling, bring your left knee toward your forehead.
74 Gently raise your head and kick your left leg backward.

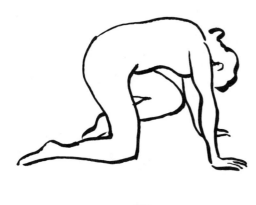

73

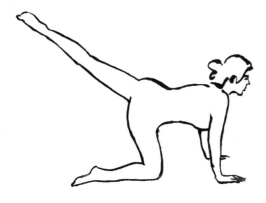

74

75 Keeping your left leg up, slowly flex your knee and foot.
76 Extend, pointing your toes.
77 Bring your left knee back to the floor.

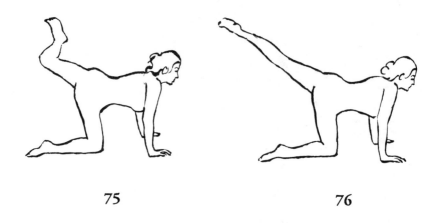

75   76

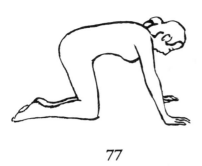

77

78 Slide your hands and shift your weight forward, bringing your pelvis and abdomen in contact with the floor. Your arms support your upper torso and your head is up.

79 Push yourself backward and sit on your heels, chest on your lap and head to the floor with arms relaxed in front of you.

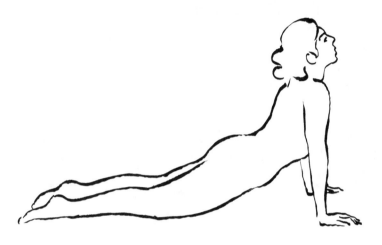

78

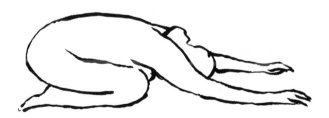

79

80 Slowly slide your arms down your sides until they lie, palms up, along your thighs. Hold this posture for about 30 seconds until you achieve a sense of peace and quiet breathing. Pay attention to the position of your neck in relation to your spine and head. Are you centered?

81 Roll up into a sitting position.

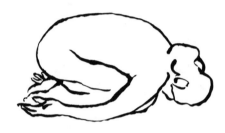

80

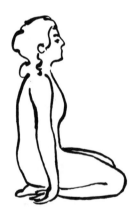

81

82 Shift your weight forward and place both palms down in front of your knees on the floor.

83 Curl your toes under you, then push yourself back into a squatting position, head down. Your hands slide toward you.

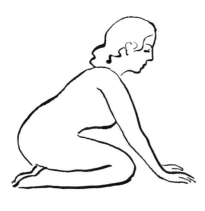

82

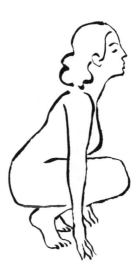

83

84 Keeping your head down and pushing with your hands, slowly drop your heels and straighten your legs. Your torso is now bent from your waist down, your heels flat on the floor, your arms relaxed.

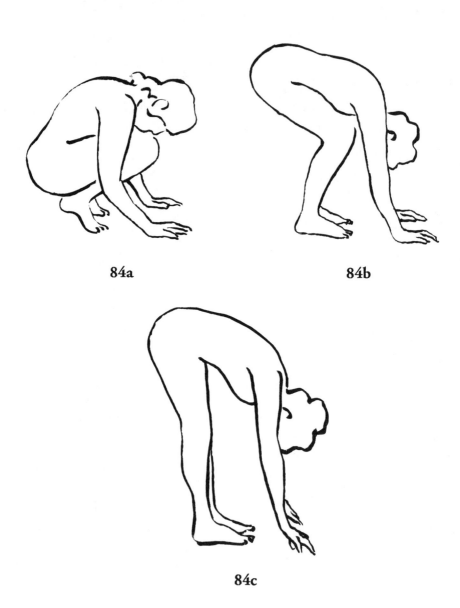

84a

84b

84c

85 Lock your thumbs. With your head nestled in the cradle of your outstretched arms, raise your arms and roll your spine up slowly. Feel each muscle as the back uncurls sensuously from the bottom up.

86 With arms above your head, inhale as you slowly arch your back, then relax.

87 Centering yourself, relax your elbows and gently lower your arms to your sides.

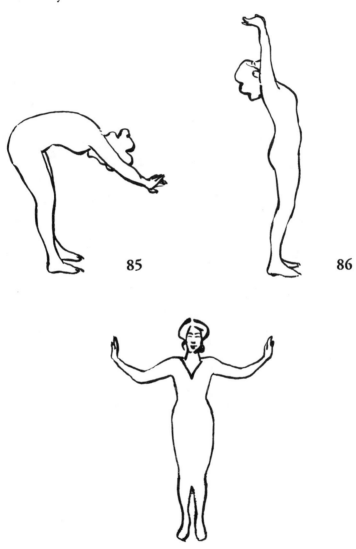

85

86

87

88 Join your hands in front of your heart and slowly bow your head. Give thanks for the day. The end is in the beginning—this is where you started!

Repeat the Dance as many times as you want. Enjoy!

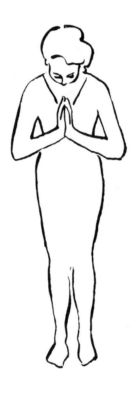

STEP NINE
Meditation

Have you ever heard someone being accused of looking at her navel? Or heard someone reply caustically after being admonished for laziness, "I was contemplating my navel." I recall when "looking at your navel" was my favorite insult. The navel to us kids was analogous to self-centeredness and selfishness. Looking at your navel was equated with showing contempt for the world!

Since then I have acquired much respect for this part of our anatomy. The umbilical cord, which passes vital fluids from mother to unborn child, is our first support system. The navel could be deemed a monument to life. It is a reminder of our vulnerability and our connection to the mystery of life.

The navel area is biologically of vital importance. Press with your index finger or thumb four points—one inch under and above, to the right and left of your navel. You are stimulating the digestive process by attracting more blood flow to the duodenum, or first 12 inches of your digestive tract.

Looking at one's navel was considered an insult in my youth. The western world was caught up in progress, technology and rational thinking. Oriental philosophy, one of the tenets of which was quiet contemplation, did not fit in with the current trend of thought. Westerners did not understand that we must try to discover the relationship between our brilliant minds and our own inner nature. When we disregard the roots of our relationship to the earth, we set for ourselves a course of doom. No amount of technology or brain research will help us unravel the mysteries of life unless we turn within, into the uncharted depths of the God within.

How does that happen? Through meditation. When you meditate, your attention turns inward to your center. The practice of meditation, rather than making you feel self-absorbed, helps you feel at peace within yourself and eventually, in harmony with the rest of the world. You cannot hope for peace in the world if you do not experience it within. Meditation helps you to focus on your different selves—physical, mental, emotional and spiritual—which leads to self-integration. Meditation liberates the inner voice—that guardian who consoles, comforts and guides your creativity.

There are as many ways to meditate as there are ways to find self-enlightenment. Do not be distracted by the variety. Judge the substance of their message, and trust that you will be guided to what is right for you. If it brings you to a closer relationship with the divine within, it is okay.

The two methods which I have followed for many years and which I find most rewarding are Zazen, or the sitting practice of Zen Buddhism (which is simply clearing the mind) and Tuning to the Higher Self.

Practice Lab: Clearing Your Mind

A Chinese proverb goes, "You cannot fill a glass with pure water if it is already half full." If your mind is half full, you cannot hear your inner voice. And in the Bible, the Book of Luke, Chapter 14, Verse 33 says, "So also none of you can be a disciple of mine without parting with all his possessions." Until you part with your distracting thoughts, you will not feel whole. Those thousand thoughts that pull you in different directions are what prevent you from being one with the divine self within. Shunryu Suzuki wrote in his book, Zen Mind, Beginner's Mind, "There is a big mind and a little mind. Little mind brings duality and pain. Big mind is Universal Nature." Zen students sit in the lotus position or sit Japanese style (on their heels or in a chair).

Sit down on a chair. Make yourself comfortable, maintaining a straight back with middle chest gently pulled up from the waist. Rest your left hand, palm open, on your lap. Your right hand, palm open, rests inside your left hand. The tips of both thumbs touch each other lightly. This hand position is referred to as *mudra* in Sanskrit. The left hand represents the passive, yielding feminine, or the yin aspect of your nature. It balances the right hand, which is the active, aggressive yang, or masculine, aspect of your nature. Together they form a union of both principles, yin and yang.

Focus your attention on your breathing. Empty your mind of all thoughts. With your mind centered, you are going to follow your breath. As you breathe in through your nose, feel the breath open your abdomen. As you breathe out, slowly count one until you release all the breath. On the next inbreath, experience the breath; and on the outbreath say *two* as you exhale. Continue until you reach 10, then return to one. There is no rush.

Seems simple, doesn't it? Why isn't it? Because a thousand

thoughts are going to assail you. "What am I going to cook for dinner tonight? How will I explain to my boss that my report is late?" What do you do with these distracting thoughts? Catch yourself in the act of thinking. Say *stop*, drop your thoughts and go right back to the count of one, empty-minded again with your sole focus being your breath.

When you get to 10, start over. You may find that you never get to count to 10. Don't struggle. What counts is the discipline you develop when you become aware of the stream of your thoughts and you release them. You will, with persistence, eventually experience a wonderful feeling of peace when you meditate that will carry into your everyday activities.

Practice about ten minutes every day in the beginning. After a week or so, extend your practice to 15 minutes, then 20. Within a short time, you will find that you are able to meditate for 30 minutes.

Practice Lab: Tuning to the Higher Self

It is probably part of your belief system that you use your will in everyday life. However, in the Ancient Mysteries, human beings are viewed as sleepwalking through life; they are in a dormant state. At this stage of our evolution, there are divine forces at work guiding us to Divine Will, which of course, supersedes the small human will. One way to become awakened to this possibility is through meditation.

What is Divine or Spiritual Will? It is Will that has its roots in absolute Wisdom. It arises out of the depth of your inner consciousness. Human beings have to recapture their divine union with the God within, the Universal principle which is all love, all goodness, all harmony and truth which permeates all creation. Each of us contains the mystery of the divine principle, the higher self. The attunement with your higher self has to be willed by you, and this is accomplished through meditation.

Practice Lab: Divine Light

Sit comfortably on a chair. Place your hands in your lap. Allow a few minutes to feel fully relaxed and attentive to your breath. When you inhale, the breath enters your inner world. When you exhale, breath is released into the outer world. In truth, there is only one breath, there is only one world.

Imagine a ball of divine light a few inches above your head. It radiates love, wisdom, harmony, clarity and life. Concentrate on its radiance for a few minutes, and become a part of it. [pause]

Feel its warmth envelop you. Imagine the ball of divine light moving down through the crown and radiating inside your head. Feel the warmth. It illuminates the sixth chakra located between your eyes. [pause]

It moves further down your throat. Feel every cell in the throat open to the warmth of that light. [pause]

From there rays of light reach out to your heart. Your heart is like a beam of light. [pause]

The light spreads further down to your solar plexus or third chakra. Every nerve is nurtured by warmth, radiance and love. [pause]

Now it moves downward to the second chakra located just below the navel. [pause]

Finally, it reaches the first chakra at the base of your spine. [pause]

From there, feel the warmth permeate your entire being. Imagine the center of each of the millions of cells that form your being pulsating with divine light. [pause]

Bring your attention to your heart center where the light is brighter than ever. Feel its radiance. Become a part of it. [pause]

From within your heart center, say these words: "In the center of my being is my divine self. It is all love, wisdom and harmony. This is my true self. It is the wisdom of pure creation. It is the essence of my being now. In this divine light, in this love, we are all united."

Allow each word to vibrate its meaning through and through. Stay immersed in the experience as long as you can. You are attuned to your Higher Self.

Practice Lab: World Peace Meditation

Thursday night is often designated by prayer groups throughout the world as an evening of spiritual study. The first such group I belonged to was called The Cathedral of the Soul. I lived in France during that period and it didn't matter whether a group was on Greenwich time or South Pacific time.

What did it matter was that like minds were gathered together on a specific day with the purpose of creating a positive vibration or thought form? Tremendous positive power can be collected in a thought form, the vibration of which can be felt around the world. When you are meditating, time and space do not count. The present moment is all there is. When you concentrate in your heart of hearts with the purpose of healing yourself or others or sending blessings to the world, what counts is the clarity of your intention and your concentration.

The following meditation offers you a way to connect with others who have the same purpose:

Choose a special place in your home or apartment where you feel relaxed. Light a candle. Sit in front of the candle and watch the flame for awhile. When it starts to dance a little, you know that you are at one with your concentration.

Close your eyes. Feel your heart beaming with divine light. Image that candle in your heart. Divine light is all warmth, love and peace. Peace enters your entire being. [pause]

From your heart center, imagine the divine light flowing into your home and with it the feeling of peace. The divine light floods the building. Feel the peace in your building. [pause]

Divine light radiates throughout your town or city. Peace surrounds your city. [pause]

Divine light enters your state or province. Peace pervades throughout the state. [pause]

Divine light expands throughout your country, bringing peace to every corner of the country. [pause]

Divine light embraces the continent, north and south, spreading peace everywhere. To the east and west, to North, Central and South America, to Europe, Africa, the Middle East; to Central Europe, the Far East, Australia and all the Pacific Islands, divine light brings its message of peace and love. Every continent, every ocean, every organism joins in a song of peace, the vibrations of which spread throughout the universe. [pause]

Look at the beautiful blue earth as though you were seeing it from a satellite. Imagine a world vibrant with love and harmony, and millions of humans and animals in perfect health with joy in their hearts. Animals, plants and minerals interact in complete harmony. All this love vibrates deep within the earth until it becomes one brilliant ball of gold. [pause]

Feel a special feeling of reverence for Mother Earth. Divine light envelopes the earth. Beams of gold spread to the solar system. Our galaxy is soon resplendent like a beaming jewel. Love, peace, and harmony are forever expanding into the universe. Open your eyes. God bless you.

Summary

Meditation is achieved through silence and concentration. It integrates your different selves—physical, emotional, mental and spiritual. In accordance with natural law, you need to clear your mind before you can tune to the little voice inside, your higher self.

Your Higher Self is the divine principle within you which needs nurturing. World Peace is a goal we all share. Let us tune to the same love vibration for our fellow man, Mother Earth and the Universe in celebration of a world where all can co-exist peacefully.

Thought for the Day

If all people around the world joined hands, one huge circle of love would form around the earth.

CHART YOUR PROGRESS

Week 1:   Tune-up

Week 2:   Tune-up plus Workout, Section A

Week 3:   Workout, Sections A and B

Week 4:   Workout, Sections A, B and C

Week 5:   Tune-up, Three Bridges and The Dance

Week 6:   Daily—The Dance

Week 7 on: Daily—The Dance
Weekly—Tune-up plus Workout, Sections A, B and C

About the Author

Katia de Peyer studied ballet at a very young age in Paris where her dance mates included Leslie Caron and Brigitte Bardot. She continued her studies in London with Madame Rambert and in Los Angeles at the School of American Ballet. She subsequently went to Madrid to study flamenco with La Quica and Mercedes y Albano, dancing professionally in Europe before moving to the United States to study dance therapy. Having successfully conducted a Ladies' Class at Carita in Paris, she offered her talents to health and glamour-conscious New Yorkers. Katia was one of the first to organize exercise classes in people's homes, which she taught in New York for twenty years, One of her many clients, Diane Von Furstenberg, asked her in the early seventies to write a special chapter on exercise in her book, *Diane Von Furstenburg's Book of Beauty.*

Her interest in Zen, in sensing awareness and healing combine with her many years of experience to make Katia's teaching intuitive and vibrant. Every summer she goes to Europe with her husband, clarinetist Gervase de Peyer, to teach a course designed to relieve the stress associated with music performance. Katia's workshop "Healing Self" has been received enthusiastically in New York and Washington. She is also at work on a project which offers healing support to people with cancer. Katia is a Reiki and MariEl practitioner.

INDEX

Some people, no matter what you give them, still want the Moon.

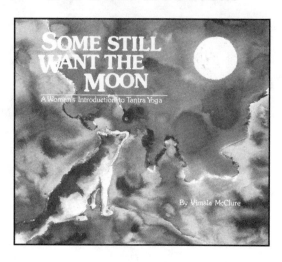

"A simple to follow instruction book on personal development using the principles and practices of Tantra Yoga. Author Vimala McClure has introduced a gentle and beautiful path for women in which all of life is spiritualized."
—Leading Edge Review

Includes:

Consciousness	Sexuality
Meditation	Pregnancy and birth
Kundalini and cakras	Diet
Yoga postures	Breathing and relaxation
Visualization and affirmation	Beauty secrets of the yogis

Plus— an illustrated step-by-step daily exercise routine.

Available from NUCLEUS Publications
Rt. 2 Box 49
Willow Springs, MO 65793
Order toll-free 1 800 762-6595
$9.95 plus $2.50 shipping. Order SM 605.

The NUCLEUS Catalog

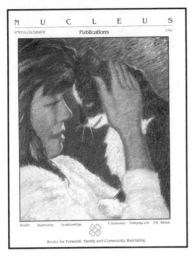

A source of inspiration:

Order these and other great books from NUCLEUS Publications.
Or ask for a free copy of our catalog.

_____ BS600 **Beyond the Superconscious Mind.** $4.95, 90 pp. by Ananda Mitra. Based on the Tantric concept of the "layers of the mind," this book explores both eastern and western understanding of how the mind works, including desire, recollection and reflection, intuition, paranormal phenomena, and meditation. A readable synthesis of research, stories, and instruction.

_____WT607 **Yoga, the Way of Tantra**. $5.95, 92 pp. Ananda Marga Publications. A general introduction to Tantra yoga; diet and health, yoga postures, meditation, ethical conduct, and philosophy.

_____ YF315 **Yoga for Health.** $5.95, 117 pp. by Ananda Mitra. This introductory book has lots of good information on the effects of yoga postures on the body and mind. Included are chapters on the glandular system and emotions, the muscles, joints, spine, circulation, internal organs. It gives clear instructions on how to perform various postures, how to breathe properly, how to do deep relaxation and self-massage, and includes an introduction to meditation.

_____ W3314 **What's Wrong With Eating Meat?** $2.50, 63 pp. by Vistara Parham. Are you interested in exploring a vegetarian or semi-vegetarian lifestyle? Are you a vegetarian with friends or relatives who question you? This is a very popular little book that reveals simply and in a straightforward manner why a vegetarian lifestyle is good for you and for the planet.

_____VL516 **The Vegetarian Lunchbasket.** $10.95, 200 pp. by Linda Haynes. Forget boring brown-bag lunches forever! Make great dinners everybody wants for lunch the next day! Linda Haynes shows you how with breads, spreads, soups, sandwiches, salads, dressings, condiments, main dishes, and desserts.

It's quick and easy to order toll-free! Call today 1-800-762-6595